Non Invasive Artificial Ventilation

T0190298

Stefano Nava · Francesco Fanfulla

Non Invasive Artificial Ventilation

How, When and Why

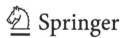 Springer

Stefano Nava
Respiratory and Critical Care Unit
AO Sant' Orsola Malpighi Hospital
Alma Mater University
Bologna
Italy

Francesco Fanfulla
Sleep Medicine Unit
Fondazione Salvatore Maugeri
Pavia
Italy

ISBN 978-88-470-5525-4   ISBN 978-88-470-5526-1   (eBook)
DOI 10.1007/978-88-470-5526-1
Springer Milan Heidelberg New York Dordrecht London

Library of Congress Control Number: 2013950738

This is the English version of the Italian edition published under the title Ventilazione meccanica non invasiva—come, quando e perché, by Stefano Nava and Francesco Fanfulla.
© Springer-Verlag Italia 2010
Translation by Rachel Stenner.
The translation of this work was funded by SEPS Segretariato Europeo per le Traduzioni Scientifiche
Via Val d'Aposa 7, 40123 Bologna, Italy. seps@seps.it, www.seps.it.

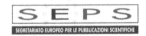

Printed on acid-free paper

Springer is part of Springer Science+Business Media (www.springer.com)

Contents

Why I Ventilate a Patient Non Invasively

1

We will start by answering a simple question. What characterizes the acute respiratory failure that best responds to non invasive ventilation (NIV)? Certainly, as shown in Fig. 1.1, one characteristic is the presence of hypercapnia and, therefore, an impairment in the respiratory pump, which comprises the central nervous system, peripheral nerves, and the respiratory muscles.

A pump deficit always leads to hypercapnia and, when not compensated, to acidosis through the mechanism of alveolar hypoventilation. This is described as the condition in which the tidal volume of gas that enters and leaves the lungs (minute volume) is no longer sufficient to meet the metabolic requirements of the body. In contrast to patients with compensated or so-called chronic respiratory acidosis, hypercapnic individuals cannot achieve a balance between the metabolic production of CO_2 and its elimination.

In simple words, for the same minute ventilation (respiratory rate × tidal volume), alveolar ventilation could be completely different. Let's consider the case of patient A, who breathes at a rate of 10 breaths/min with a tidal volume of 500 mL, and that of patient B, who breathes at a rate of 20 breaths/min with a tidal volume of 250 mL. Both have the same minute ventilation (5 L/min), but they have completely different values of alveolar ventilation. If the dead space in the two patients is the same, for example 150 mL, the alveolar ventilation in the former patient is 3.5 L/min (500−150 mL = 350 mL × 10 breaths/min) while that in the latter is 2 L/min (250−150 mL = 100 mL × 20 breaths/min). It is this respiratory pattern, characterized by breathing that is rapid (high respiratory rates) and shallow (low tidal volumes), which leads to the development of hypercapnia.

The diagnosis of acute, hypercapnic respiratory failure is based above all on values of PaO_2 (otherwise what respiratory failure would it be?) <60 mmHg in room air and $PaCO_2$ > 45–50 mmHg with a pH < 7.35.

These formal limits do not, however, take into consideration numerous factors, the foremost being the time variable, as well as the way the episode developed and the age of the patient. For example, a $PaCO_2$ of 70 mmHg that develops over several weeks has a different significance from the same value reached in a few hours, so our diagnosis must be based on the pH (or degree of compensation).

S. Nava and F. Fanfulla, *Non Invasive Artificial Ventilation*,
DOI: 10.1007/978-88-470-5526-1_1, © Springer-Verlag Italia 2014

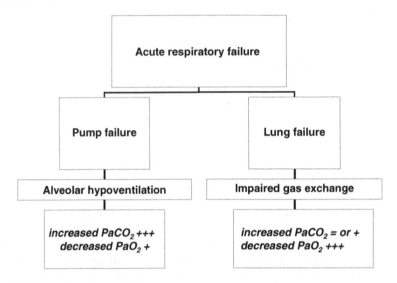

Fig. 1.1 Types of respiratory failure

In most cases, NIV is able to return our patients' blood-gas values to more appropriate, even if not completely normal, levels by correcting the respiratory pattern, that is, by increasing the tidal volume with the help of the ventilator and at the same time reducing the respiratory rate. In patients with chronic obstructive pulmonary disease (COPD), this latter effect also has the result of giving the individuals more time to exhale and, thereby, reduces the degree of dynamic hyperinflation.

The pathophysiology of purely hypoxic respiratory failure is more complex and depends of various factors, not all of which involve the lungs, such as cardiocirculatory failure. However, the most common changes in the so-called respiratory failure of parenchymal origin are those in the ventilation/perfusion ratio, shunt, and diffusion.

The classical definition of acute respiratory failure is based on a $PaO_2/FiO_2 < 300$, with increasing severity as the value of this ratio decreases. In these forms of respiratory failure, NIV is often not as effective as invasive ventilation which is, therefore, preferred as the first-line treatment, at least in some cases, for questions of safety. The reasons why intubation is often used are well-known:

- to protect the airways;
- because of the need for continuous ventilation and, therefore, sedation and sometimes even neuromuscular blockade;
- severe hemodynamic instability;
- use of high fractions of inspired oxygen, which is sometimes not possible with non invasive ventilators.

There are, however, conditions characterized by hypoxic respiratory failure which respond very well to NIV, particularly acute pulmonary edema and pneumonia in immunocompromised subjects (these conditions are discussed later in specific chapters).

Suggested Reading

Bégin P, Grassino A (1991) Inspiratory muscle dysfunction and chronic hypercapnia in chronic obstructive pulmonary disease. Am Rev Resp Dis 143:905–912

Bellemare F, Grassino A (1983) Force reserve of the diaphragm in patients with chronic obstructive pulmonary disease. J Appl Physiol 55:8–15

Ceriana P, Nava S (2006) Hypoxic and hypercapnic respiratory failure. In: Nava S, Welte T (eds) Respiratory emergencies (European respiratory monograph). European Respiratory Society Journals Ltd, Sheffield

Moloney ED, Kiely JL, McNicholas WT (2001) Controlled oxygen therapy and carbon dioxide retention during exacerbations of chronic obstructive pulmonary disease. Lancet 357(9255):526–528

NHLBI Workshop summary (1990) Respiratory muscle fatigue: report of the respiratory muscle fatigue workshop group. Am Rev Respir Dis 142(2):474–480

Similowski T, Yan S, Gauthier AP et al (1991) Contractile properties of the human diaphragm during chronic hyperinflation. N Engl J Med 325(13):917–923

Stevenson NJ, Walker PP, Costello RW, Calverley PM (2005) Lung mechanics and dyspnea during exacerbations of chronic obstructive pulmonary disease. Am J Respir Crit Care Med 172(12):1510–1516

The Physiology of Mechanical Ventilation

2

The aim of this chapter is to try to describe, briefly and simply, the basics of how a ventilator works and provide some notions on the interaction between the ventilator and the patient.

A ventilator is a relatively simple machine designed to transmit and apply, following a set scheme, energy which serves to perform useful work. The energy is delivered to the ventilator in the form of electricity (= volts × amperes × time) or compressed gas (= pressure × volume) and conveyed from it in order to increase or replace the force that the respiratory muscles must expend to support the work of breathing.

However, let's take a step backwards and try to understand how we breathe. First of all, we have to define what must be translated from pure mechanics to respiratory physiology. Force is a mechanical concept that in physiology is defined as pressure (pressure = force/area), movement is the volume (volume = area × movement), and finally the measure of the change in movement is defined as flow (mean flow = Δ volume/Δ time). In the case of ventilation, we consider a pressure generated by a subject and/or by a machine which produces a flow of gas that enters the airways and increases the volume of the lungs.

Figure 2.1 is a diagram showing, simply we hope, how breathing works. To begin with there are three pressures that determine the flow and, therefore, the generation of volume; these are:

1. the atmospheric pressure (Patm);
2. the alveolar pressure, that is, the pressure within the lungs (Palv);
3. the pleural pressure, that is, the pressure generated between the lungs and the thoracic cage (Ppl).

The movement of air from outside the body into the lungs and vice versa is ensured by a pressure gradient between the exterior (Patm) and interior of the lungs (Palv). If the Palv decreases, with respect to the Patm, we talk of negative pressure ventilation, which is the natural condition. If the Patm (pressure at the mouth) increases, with respect to the Palv, we talk of positive pressure ventilation

S. Nava and F. Fanfulla, *Non Invasive Artificial Ventilation*,
DOI: 10.1007/978-88-470-5526-1_2, © Springer-Verlag Italia 2014

Fig. 2.1 How the respiratory
system works

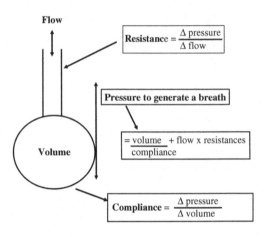

(during mechanical ventilation). The greater the flow, the greater the pressure; as a
corollary, for the same flow, if the resistance increases, the pressure rises.

The expansion of an elastic balloon is caused by the so-called transpulmonary
pressure, that is, the difference between Palv and Ppl. The force that generates a
breath is produced during mechanical ventilation by the sum of the pressure of the
patient's muscles (Pmusc) and the pressure generated by the ventilator (Pvent).

Two other pressures are important in determining the physiology of a spontaneous or an assisted breath: the pressure of elastic recoil (i.e., elastance or $E = \Delta$
pressure/Δ volume, with compliance being its reciprocal), and the resistive pressure (i.e., $R = \Delta$ pressure/Δ flow), which depends on the patient's characteristics.
In the final analysis, the so-called equation of motion of the respiratory system can
be simplified as follows:

$$P_{vent} + P_{musc} = \text{Elastance} \times \text{Volume} + \text{Resistance} \times \text{Flow}$$

Thus, in the ventilated patient, the pressures generated by the ventilator and the
patient, in various proportions depending on the pathology and the method of
ventilation, determine the flow and volume that the patient receives. For example,
a totally passive patient has no Pmusc and so all the force is generated by Pvent;
the opposite condition exists if the patient is breathing spontaneously.

Pressure, volume, and flow are functions of time and are called *variables*. It is
assumed that elastance and resistances remain constant during breathing and, by
convention, these are called *parameters*. This applies to the inspiratory phase.

Supposing that expiration occurs passively, as it does in the majority of cases,
Pmusc and Pvent are absent and the equation of motion therefore becomes:

$$-\text{Resistance} \times \text{Flow} = \text{Elastance} \times \text{Volume}$$

The minus sign at the left of the equation indicates the negative direction of the
expiratory flow and suggests that during passive expiration the flow is generated

by the energy stored in the elastic component during inspiration. These are the basic concepts that we must keep in mind when we ventilate a patient, remembering that probably the only difference between invasive ventilation and NIV is given by the resistance of the nose and the upper airway, which are by-passed by the endotracheal tube in invasive ventilation.

Suggested Reading

Bates JH, Rossi A, Milic-Emili J (1985) Analysis of the behaviour of the respiratory system with constant inspiratory flow. J Appl Physiol 58(6):1840–1848

Chatburn RL (2006) Classification of mechanical ventilators. In: Tobin M (ed) Principle and practice of mechanical ventilation. Mc-Graw Hill, New York

Mead J, Lindgren I, Gaensler EA (1955) The mechanical properties of the lungs in emphysema. J Clin Invest 34:1005–1016

(Almost) Everything You Wanted to Know About a Ventilator

3

NIV is no longer delivered exclusively by the so-called "home" ventilators, but by a broad selection of machines ranging from sophisticated and expensive intensive care ventilators to those used for home care. For this reason we have divided the ventilators into broad categories, taking into account that the severity of the patient's condition, the acuteness of the respiratory failure, and the timing and setting in which the NIV is used also determine the choice of ventilator, the interface, and disposables. Furthermore, it should be appreciated that, given the continuous technological improvements, many ventilator models are modified or even replaced within just a few months.

The first ventilators for NIV used a method of volume-controlled ventilation or synchronized intermittent mandatory ventilation (SIMV), while only some of them also offered the option of pressure-controlled ventilation. These machines did their work very well for about 30 years, ventilating thousands of patients at home, mostly in an invasive manner but also, in some cases, non invasively; however, the main limitation to the use of these ventilators in a non invasive manner was their fixed pattern of delivering the inspired gas, making them incapable of compensating for the inevitable air losses, as well as the fact that an extrinsic PEEP (PEEPe) value could not be set for some of them.

The "generational change" that gave rise to the modern pressure ventilators derived from a continuous positive airway pressure (CPAP) ventilator used for the treatment of nocturnal apnea, to which a magnetic valve was applied so that two different levels of pressure could be delivered during inspiration and expiration. This gave rise to the name "*bilevel positive airway* pressure." The success of this ventilator, and other similar models that quickly entered the market, lay in its reduced weight and bulk, its easy portability, simplicity of use, and in the possibility of eliminating the alarms, which are often not necessary in patients who are not dependent on the ventilator.

The technological progress made in the last 20 years has meant that there is now a range of ventilators on the market which have been specifically designed for NIV and whose performance does not differ greatly from that of the ventilators for intensive care. This large variety of ventilators now available on the market does

S. Nava and F. Fanfulla, *Non Invasive Artificial Ventilation*,
DOI: 10.1007/978-88-470-5526-1_3, © Springer-Verlag Italia 2014

not always make it easy to classify them within precise classes since many of them, as indicated above, are "hybrid" models. Having said this, for the sake of simplicity we have divided the ventilators into four main classes:

• Intensive care ventilators with an NIV module;
• Intensive care ventilators specific for NIV;
• Simple and/or home bilevel ventilators;
• Stand-alone CPAP.

3.1   How a Ventilator Works

Here below we try to simplify some of the basic concepts regarding how a ventilator works, which are often misunderstood by the "general public".

The task of a ventilator is to transform energy into one of the output variables, such as flow, pressure, or volume. This can be achieved by applying a positive pressure to the airways or a subatmospheric pressure to the exterior of the chest, as in the case of negative pressure ventilation.

Schematically a ventilator can be classified as pressure, volume, flow, and time controlled. From a practical point of view it is useful to keep the following rules in mind:

• if the pressure signal is not altered when the mechanical properties of the patient change, the ventilator is *pressure* controlled;
• if the volume delivered is measured directly by the ventilator, then the ventilator is *volume* controlled;
• if the volume delivered is determined by a flow transducer, the ventilator is *flow*-cycled;
• if the flow and volume signals are altered following changes in resistances and compliance, the ventilator is *time*-controlled.

The most commonly used ventilators are, of course, those cycled by volume or pressure. Ventilators require a source of electricity, which may be an alternating current (AC), or direct current (DC) when battery-powered.

3.1.1   Pressurized Gas System

The source of gas may be an external gas at high pressure, as in the case of a centralized delivery system, an internal compressor, turbine or a piston, or a hybrid system.

Simplifying the matter, a ventilator with a NIV option can work with oxygen and air at high pressure (i.e., 4 atmospheres) or oxygen and air at atmospheric pressure.

In the former category of machine, typically present in Intensive Care Units, the pressure within the ventilator is reduced to atmospheric level in order to allow the patient to breathe physiologically. The peak flow delivered is usually very fast, reaching >200 L/m and the flow is maintained constant at a level of 130–150 L/m.

In the latter category of ventilator, to which most of the ventilators designed specifically for NIV belong, the piston or a turbine aspirates air from the atmosphere. The simultaneous use of oxygen at a high flow rate means that these machines can also be useful in the Intensive Care Unit. The peak flow exceeds 200 L/m considerably, but, particularly in the oldest ventilators, the application of resistance can lead to a dramatic reduction in flow to values even below <100 L/ m. Fast turbines or turbines that rotate at a constant velocity regulated by a proportional valve have enabled the latest generation ventilators to perform equally well as those fed with oxygen and air at high pressure. These machines can very often meet the ventilatory requirements of patients in respiratory distress.

Some turbine-based home ventilators have the option of being able to enrich the system only with oxygen at a low flow (from a cylinder or the classical hospital flow meter), but in this case the pressure of the gas is not constant.

3.1.2 Source of Gas

The ventilators in both categories very frequently include an internal blender guided by a proportional valve. Some ventilators that work with room air do not have a real and proper blender, but an oxygen-delivering system consisting of a proportional valve that combines the air sucked in by the turbine.

3.1.3 Inspiratory and Expiratory Valves

The main task of the two valves is to regulate the respiratory cycle and in particular to control the beginning and the end of the inspiratory phase. In most ventilators the inspiratory valve is regulated by an on–off system, or by a proportional valve (typically solenoid) which opens and closes in proportion to the flow, potentially keeping the circuit open all the time.

The expiratory valve can, therefore, work with an open-close mechanism, in alternation with the inspiratory valve (a typical "mushroom" o "diaphragm" valve), or with proportional opening, as described above. The expiratory valves also determine the pressure of the system during the expiratory phase, at atmospheric level or maintaining a positive expiratory pressure (external PEEP).

Solenoid valves or microprocessors that regulate the expiratory valve are useful in order to reduce the expiratory time constants, particularly in patients with limited flow. In some ventilators and modalities the so-called expiratory valves can be kept active at all times: this enables the patient to breathe spontaneously during a pressure-controlled breath (i.e., APRV or BiPAP).

3.1.4 Inspiratory and Expiratory Triggers

The reader is referred to the chapters on ventilator settings.

3.1.5 Alarms

Almost all ventilators have "absolute" safety alarms that cannot be deactivated by the operator, since their silencing could put the patient's health at risk. The alarms in this category are those related to failure of the electrical current, apnea, FiO_2, and high pressure, this last usually being placed between the inspiratory and expiratory valve and acting automatically to eliminate any excess pressure in the ventilator circuit. An interesting option of some ventilators with a NIV mode is the differentiation of the alarm for real disconnection from that of massive air loss because of poor positioning of the interface. The most common alarms that the operator can modify are those related to the pressure, volume, frequency, and ventilation/minute.

3.1.6 The Monitoring System

The presence or absence of a monitoring system does not directly affect the patient's safety, but it certainly helps the operator to interpret the patient's clinical course better.

During NIV, it is definitely important to be able to see the values of the tidal volume, which we remind you, are calculated as the integral of the flow signal. The expiratory volume is essential in order to control the efficacy of the mechanical ventilation. The difference between the inspired volume and the expired volume is useful for quantifying the presence of losses of the system during NIV. There are ventilators that measure the two volumes (i.e., inspiratory and expiratory) directly and others that extrapolate them from the flow signal and from the losses. The true measure of the two volumes can only be obtained with two pneumotachographs placed on the inspiratory and expiratory limbs, or with one pneumotachograph introduced at the Y of a double-tube system. The technical data sheet of each ventilator includes information on the ventilator's monitoring system.

Fortunately, ventilators that determined the volume exclusively from the inspiratory flow, without taking into consideration any losses, have almost completely disappeared from the market. Indeed, in this case the ventilator algorithm tried to compensate by increasing the inspiratory flow, thereby directly influencing the reading of the volume, which became abnormally higher the greater the losses were. We found numbers which indicated volumes even greater than a liter, when perhaps the real tidal volume was only a few tens of milliliters. For many years this led to confusion.

Although pressure-preset NIV is able to compensate for nonintentional leaks better than volume-preset NIV, a constant tidal volume may not be guaranteed in the presence of changes in respiratory impedance. To overcome this problem, a volume-guaranteed (VTG) mode has recently been introduced in most bilevel ventilators both in double-limb and in single-limb circuits. The ability of the VTG mode to compensate for nonintentional leaks depends however strictly on whether a "vented" (i.e., nonrebreathing valve) or "non-vented" (true expiratory valves) circuit configuration is used. This difference must be taken into account as a possible risk when a VTG mode is used with a "non-vented" circuit (see also in the next chapter for further details).

Flow, pressure, and volume traces have become very popular in recent years; in our opinion their real value is directly proportional to the pathophysiological knowledge of the operator. These curves are very useful for visualizing the patient-ventilator interaction and the characteristics of the expiratory flow. In the invasively ventilated patient, in whom deep sedation and/or neuromuscular blockade is possible, the values of the mechanical respiration can be measured directly (for example, compliance, resistance, static intrinsic PEEP) through occlusion maneuvers at end inspiration and expiration.

3.1.7 Comparative Studies

We don't want to be part of the 'politically correct' and, therefore, often hypo-critical herd and state here that, although there have been giant steps forward in technology and almost all the available ventilators are reliable and safe, there are important differences between ventilators in the same category. First of all we want to belie the common belief that critical care ventilators are necessarily more sophisticated and "perform better" only because they cost more and have more elaborate monitoring. We should remember that a ventilator for NIV must, by principle, have complex algorithms to compensate for losses. This said, various studies have now been published comparing the performance of a variety of machines *in vitro*, although almost never *in vivo*. We invite the reader to analyze the studies cited at the end of this chapter to discover the reliability of inspiratory and expiratory triggering systems, the effort required by the patients and last, but not least, the ease of use. In this regards, we want to report the findings of Gonzalez-Bermejo (Gonzalez-Bermejo et al. 2006), who demonstrated that, for the same operator, the time needed to start a ventilator varies between 20 and 120 s depending on the type of machine used. You should also remember that the presence of losses significantly influences the performance of a ventilator.

Furthermore, if and when you read published studies, you should appreciate that: (1) they are often already "old" when they are published, since the algorithms in some of the ventilators could have been changed or the ventilators have been replaced by new models; (2) extrapolation of *in vitro* findings to patients may not be appropriate; and (3) the tests carried out to verify the efficacy of the compensation of losses are often performed with predetermined values (usually moderate and severe losses) whereas in real life the air that escapes can vary considerably from breath to breath.

Finally, remember that the performance of a ventilator should not be judged from reports or brochures that companies show you. For example, the flow supplied by a ventilator is not necessarily synonymous with good or poor performance; a machine can guarantee a high flow, but have you ever asked yourself for how many seconds that flow can be maintained varying, for example, the FiO_2 or the resistive component? The efficacy of a ventilator is also judged on the basis of this.

Suggested Reading

Carlucci A, Schreiber A, Mattei A, Malovini A, Bellinati J, Ceriana P, Gregoretti C (2013) The configuration of bi-level ventilator circuits may affect compensation for non-intentional leaks during volume-targeted ventilation. Intensive Care Med 39(1):59–65

Carteaux G, Lyazidi A, Cordoba-Izquierdo A, Vignaux L, Jolliet P, Thille A, Richard JC, Brochard L (2012) Patient-ventilator asynchrony during noninvasive ventilation a bench and clinical study. Chest 142(2):367–376

Gonzalez-Bermejo J, Laplanche V, Husseini FE et al (2006) Evaluation of user-friendliness of 11 home mechanical ventilators. Eur Respir J 27(6):1236–1243

Gregoretti C, Navalesi P, Tosetti I, Pelosi P (2008) How to choose an intensive care unit ventilator? The buyers' guide to respiratory care products. Available on http://www.ersbuyersguide.org/

Kaczmarek RM et al (2006) Basic principles of ventilatory machinery. In: Tobin M (ed) Principles and practice of mechanical ventilation. McGraw-Hill, New York

Mehta S, McCool FD, Hill NS (2001) Leak compensation in positive pressure ventilators: a lung model study. Eur Respir J 17(2):259–267

Richard JC, Carlucci A, Breton L et al (2002) Bench testing of pressure support ventilation with three different generations of ventilators. Intensive Care Med 28(8):1049–1057

Vignaux L, Tassaux D, Jolliet P (2007) Performance of noninvasive ventilation modes on ICU ventilators during pressure support: a bench model study. Intensive Care Med 33(8):1444–1451

Vitacca M, Barbano L, D'Anna S (2002) Comparison of five bilevel pressure ventilators in patients with chronic respiratory failure. A physiologic study. Chest 122(6):2105–2114

The Interfaces for NIV

4

The choice of the most appropriate interface is undoubtedly one of the corner-stones of the success of NIV, not only for patients with acute respiratory failure in whom the seal and efficacy are the most important features, but also in the setting of long-term ventilation, in which comfort is more important. The choice of interface is also crucial with regards to the development of side effects, such as loss of air, claustrophobia, facial erythema, acne-like rash, pressure sores, and conjunctival irritation; in confirmation of this aspect, which despite being recognized is often ignored, in a study of more than 3,000 patients receiving home ventilation with CPAP it was noted that only half of the patients considered their NIV mask satisfactory.

The interfaces can be classified as:
- oral: the only interface of this type is the mouthpiece, which is introduced between the lips and held in place by a lip seal;
- nasal: nasal masks and nasal olives; these latter, which are called 'nasal pillows' in English, are soft rubber plugs introduced into the nostrils.;
- oro-nasal: face masks (covering the nose and mouth) and full face masks (also including the eyes);
- helmet: also includes the neck, but does not come into contact with the skin of the face.

The interfaces can be manufactured industrially ready for use and distributed by different medical companies in various sizes for children and adults, or they can be made to measure, by taking a direct impression or a cast of the face.

The ready-to-use industrially made masks are usually modular and consist of two or more parts: a cushion, in direct contact with the skin, made of a soft material (PVC, polypropylene, silicone, hydro-gel, silicone elastomer, etc.) and a shell of rigid material, which is usually transparent (rigid PVC, polycarbonate, etc.); these parts can be detached and are assembled using an interlocking mechanism or are soldered together. The advantage of the modular mask is that only the cushion needs to be changed when it becomes worn out, which reduces

S. Nava and F. Fanfulla, *Non Invasive Artificial Ventilation*,
DOI: 10.1007/978-88-470-5526-1_4, © Springer-Verlag Italia 2014

the costs of maintenance. The mask has between two and eight anchorage points to which the fixation system of the mask itself is attached using hooks or strips of Velcro. The higher the number of anchorage sites, the greater the possibility of obtaining optimal fixation and of being able to vary the points of maximal pressure; the attachments are usually arranged peripherally on the mask, thereby producing a more uniform distribution of pressure on the face. The masks can have holes which act as an anti-rebreathing system; if such masks are used, the ventilator should not have a two-way circuit nor should other devices be included in a one-way circuit for the elimination of carbon dioxide (see later). Supplementary holes which may be present in the masks can serve for the administration of oxygen, for measuring the pressure at the opening of the airways or for capnometry.

The nasal bridge is usually the most delicate part and the one most at risk of reddening and pressure sores, also because of a possible individual skin intolerance to the material from which the mask is made or excessive sweating. In any case, it is essential that the mask is not fixed too tightly in order to prevent pressure sores; the general recommendation is to fix the mask in such a way that two fingers can pass between this and the face, accepting a minimal degree of air loss, if this does not interfere with the interaction between the patient and the ventilator.

An additional strategy to prevent pressure sores, if the patient has to remain non invasively ventilated for many hours consecutively, is to use different types of masks. In this way the distribution of the pressure on the skin is alternated and the points of maximum friction, especially on the bridge of the nose, are varied.

4.1   Mouthpieces

Mouthpieces are fairly widely used, particularly in the United States of America, in patients with neuromuscular disorders. They can be used as the only interface or as the interface applied during the day, alternated with another interface used during the night. Mouthpieces come in various shapes and sizes, in order to adapt to the different conformations of the oral cavity; some can be applied as dental devices so that they can be removed simply by protruding the tongue. The drawbacks of their use are stimulation of salivation and the pharyngeal reflex, to the point of inducing vomiting; their long-term use can also cause deformities of the dental arches. Aerophagy and gastric distention are more common with mouthpieces than with other types of interface.

4.2   Nasal Masks

These are used preferentially for stable patients requiring long-term home NIV or also in hospital in the case of new onset respiratory failure, once the acute phase has passed. When using such masks at home, care must be taken to check for any air leakage from the mouth, particularly during the hours of nocturnal sleep, during which the patient may not notice involuntary opening of the mouth in the absence of a system of controlling this (alarms on the inspired tidal volume or someone able to supervise the patient). This drawback can be overcome by using appropriate Velcro fixation systems (chin straps) that prevent movements of the jaw.

4.3   Nasal Pillows

This type of interface has the same advantages as nasal masks with regards to allowing the patient to expectorate, eat, and talk without removing the interface; furthermore, it causes less sensation of claustrophobia, for those who suffer from this problem, and allows the patient to wear glasses during the NIV, which is often an important aspect. It is mostly used as an alternative, at least for some hours, to a face mask or nasal mask to eliminate the problem of friction of the skin of the nose in people at high risk of developing pressure sores. In this way the tolerance of NIV can be increased and, in parallel, the number of hours of use. The advantages and disadvantages are the same as those of the nasal masks.

4.4   Face Masks

These are the interfaces of first choice for patients in acute respiratory failure who, to reduce respiratory resistance, use oro-nasal respiration.

A recent survey carried out in about 300 wards, between intensive care and respiratory wards, confirmed that face masks are the most widely used interface during episodes of acute respiratory failure, followed by nasal masks, full face masks, and helmets. The reason for this preference lies in the nurses' and/or respiratory therapists' familiarity with the use of the face mask, the patients' comfort and the lesser air leakage. In recent years, there has been remarkable technological progress with improvement of the cushion that rests on the face, mechanisms for fast attachment and detachment, as well as anti-asphyxia valves to prevent rebreathing or asphyxia if the ventilator does not work correctly. The full face masks have a soft cushion which adapts well to the contour of the face thus avoiding direct pressure on the face; the shell of the mask includes an anti-asphyxia valve which opens automatically to room air if the ventilator functions poorly when the pressure in the airways falls below 3 cmH$_2$O.

4.5   Helmets

These are cylindrical, transparent casings made of PVC, separated by a metal ring from the collar (made of PVC or silicone) which adheres to the neck providing a sealed connection and optimal airtightness. Helmets are available in different sizes.

They have two entrances, which act as inspiratory and expiratory pathways, an anti-asphyxia valve and metal pins on the anterior and posterior surfaces of the ring. These pins enable the helmet to be anchored to the patient's armpits by two padded straps. Helmets have been used for the treatment of hypoxemic and hypercapnic respiratory failure and have the advantage that direct contact between the interface and the patient's skin is avoided and so the interface can be used continuously for long periods. However, the large dead space can promote rebreathing and reduce the elimination of carbon dioxide, while the distensibility of the wall and the large internal volume of gas can affect the mechanism triggering inspiration and expiration, worsening the interaction between the patient and the machine, although there seem to be some differences in this phenomenon depending on the model of helmet used.

These features make a helmet ideal for use with CPAP, provided that it is connected to a source of fresh gas able to deliver high rates of flow above 30 L/m. The advantages and disadvantages of each class and type of interface are presented in Fig. 4.1, while some of the "myths" surrounding the use of the different types of mask (for example, those regarding the dead space and the frequency of use) are described in detail in the chapters discussing "myths" and "tips and traps".

MOUTHPIECES		NASAL CUSHIONS	
Advantages	Disadvantages	Advantages	Disadvantages
• Useful in "rotating" strategy	• Vomiting and hypersalivation • Losses • Gastric distension • Talking is difficult	• Useful in "rotating" strategy • No nasal abrasions	• V_T cannot be monitored • Losses • Nasal irritation

NASAL MASKS		FACE MASKS	
Advantages	Disadvantages	Advantages	Disadvantages
• Talking possible • Eating possible • Expectoration possible • Limited risk of vomiting • Minimal risk of asphyxia	• Losses if mouth open • Nasal abrasions • Not possible with nasal obstruction	• Reduced losses • Does not require much collaboration • Can be positioned according to patient's comfort	• Vomiting • Claustrophobia • Nasal abrasions (not with "total") • Talking and coughing are difficult

HELMETS	
Advantages	Disadvantages
• Minimal losses • Does not require much collaboration • No skin abrasions	• Rebreathing possible • Vomiting • Noisy • Asynchrony with patient • Axillary discomfort

Fig. 4.1 Pros and cons of the various interfaces

Suggested Reading

Antonelli M, Conti G, Pelosi P et al (2002) New treatment of acute hypoxemic respiratory failure: noninvasive pressure support ventilation delivered by helmet–a pilot controlled trial. Crit Care Med 30(3):602–608

Antonelli M, Pennisi MA, Pelosi P et al (2004) Noninvasive positive pressure ventilation using a helmet in patients with acute exacerbation of chronic obstructive pulmonary disease: a feasibility study. Anesthesiology 100(1):16–24

Fauroux B, Lavis JF, Nicot F (2005) Facial side effects during noninvasive positive pressure ventilation in children. Intensive Care Med 31(7):965–969

Fodil R, Lellouche F, Mancebo J, Sbirlea-Apiou G, Isabey D, Brochard L, Louis B (2011) Comparison of patient–ventilator interfaces based on their computerized effective dead space. Intensive Care Med 37:257–262

Milan M, Zanella A, Isgrò S, El Sayed Deab SAEA, Magni F, Pesenti A, Patroniti N (2011) Performance of different continuous positive airway pressure helmets equipped with safety valves during failure of fresh gas supply. Intensive Care Med 37:1031–1035

Nava S, Navalesi P, Gregoretti C (2009) Interfaces and humidification for non-invasive ventilation. Respir Care 54(1):71–84

Navalesi P, Fanfulla F, Frigerio P et al (2000) Physiologic evaluation of noninvasive mechanical ventilation delivered with three types of masks in patients with chronic hypercapnic respiratory failure. Crit Care Med 28(6):1785–1790

Ozsancak A, Sidhom SS, Liesching TN, Howard W, Hill NS (2011) Evaluation of the total face mask for noninvasive ventilation to treat acute respiratory failure. Chest 139:1034–1041

Patroniti N, Saini M, Zanella A et al (2007) A Danger of helmet continuous positive airway pressure during failure of fresh gas source supply. Intensive Care Med 33(1):153–157

Saatci E, Miller DM, Stell IM et al (2004) Dynamic dead space in face masks used with noninvasive ventilators: a lung model study. Eur Respir J 23(1):129–135

Schettino P, Tucci R, Sousa R et al (2001) Mask mechanics and leak dynamics during noninvasive pressure support ventilation: a bench study. Intensive Care Med 27(12):1887–1891

When to Start (or Not) Ventilation Treatment

5

Faced with a suffering, dyspneic patient with acute respiratory failure, we often wonder whether there are the objective conditions to start ventilation therapy. We lovers of NIV are always being asked what are the criteria for starting NIV, while I have never heard an intensive care specialist being asked what are the objective parameters for intubating a patient. There are cases in which invasive ventilation therapy is essential, such as during anesthesia, in patients with respiratory arrest of various causes, when the airways must be kept patent, in patients with a seriously compromised sensorium, and in those with very severe hypoxia. Common sense, a "clinical eye," the degree of dyspnea, worsening blood gases and, lastly, but by no means an irrelevant factor, the availability of beds, are the factors that influence the choice of the intensive care specialist when faced with a patient with severe acute respiratory failure.

5.1 The Timing of Application

On the other hand, there are fairly clear criteria on the initiation of NIV, since all the studies published in recent years have placed much emphasis on standardizing the parameters of use of NIV according to the type of respiratory failure. What has never been sufficiently emphasized, in our opinion, is the timing of application of NIV. This depends on the severity of the patients' conditions, the context in which the method is applied and, above all, our expectations regarding NIV.

In other words, we believe that there are three fundamental circumstances, indicated in Fig. 5.1, which depend on the severity of the respiratory failure and, at the same time, on the meaning we give to starting NIV.

The first circumstance is when we apply NIV to a patient in the initial stages of hypercapnic or hypoxic acute respiratory failure, when no one in the past would have considered ventilating a patient in that clinical state, or even less so, admitting him or her to the Intensive Care Unit, to *prevent* a worsening of respiratory failure.

S. Nava and F. Fanfulla, *Non Invasive Artificial Ventilation*,
DOI: 10.1007/978-88-470-5526-1_5, © Springer-Verlag Italia 2014

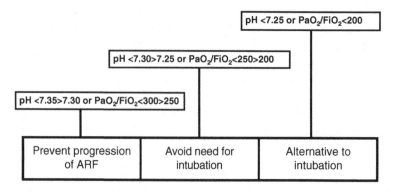

Fig. 5.1 Timing of application

The second circumstance occurs when the patient's condition is more critical and the respiratory failure is more overt, although the patient could, perhaps, still be treated outside an Intensive Care Unit with medical therapy, when the NIV is applied to *avoid* intubation.

Finally, the third circumstance, when the "going gets tough," is when a brief trial of NIV is performed in a protected environment (i.e., an Intensive or Subintensive Care Unit), with the aim of the NIV being an *alternative* to intubation.

As far as concerns the parameters to consider, analysis of arterial blood gases is essential, since it is the only investigation that enables the diagnosis of respiratory failure to be made. The other parameters serve above all to establish the severity of the patient's condition and respiratory stress.

5.2   Arterial Blood-Gas Analysis

The first information that we obtain from blood-gas analysis is whether the respiratory failure is of a hypoxic type or hypercapnic type and, in this latter case, if it is associated with respiratory acidosis.

A PaO_2/FiO_2 ratio that drops abruptly to below 300 is usually an indicator of acute respiratory failure and in such a situation there could already be the criteria for starting NIV. Of course a PaO_2 of 63 Torr in a patient with chronic respiratory disease breathing room air does not have the same significance as the same value in a 25-year old with pneumonia.

As far as regards the $PaCO_2$, the development of hypercapnia is almost always related to a defect in the respiratory pump. A value higher than 50 mmHg should be an alarm bell in every case, but it is obvious that the need to start mechanical ventilation depends on the chronicity of the disease and, therefore, on the degree of acidosis.

Table 5.1 Selection of patients

Clinical examination
Increased dyspnea
• Tachypnea (>25 breaths/min in COPD; >30 in restrictive disorders)
• Signs of increased respiratory work (e.g., use of accessory muscles and paradoxical abdominal movements)
Gas exchange
Acute on chronic respiratory failure
• $PaCO_2$ > 45 mmHg, pH < 7.35
• Hypoxia
• PaO_2/FIO_2 < 200
Contraindications
• Respiratory arrest
• Shock
• Uncontrolled cardiac arrhythmias and/or myocardial infarction
• Uncontrolled bleeding from the gastrointestinal system
• Inability to protect the airways
• Excessive secretions without being able to expectorate despite manual or mechanical aid
• Inability to apply an interface
• Recent surgery to the upper airways or upper digestive tract

As shown in Table 5.1, NIV is indicated in patients with chronic obstructive pulmonary disease (COPD) with high values of $PaCO_2$, but only in the presence of a pH < 7.35. Hypercapnia in the absence of acidosis is never a criterion for acute ventilation. The interpretation of the blood-gas values should not, of course, be limited simply to the three classical parameters described above, but should also include bicarbonates, base excess, alveolar-capillary gradient, etc., for a better understanding of the real state of the acid–base balance.

5.3 Dyspnea

This is defined in various ways as the lack of breath, difficulty in breathing, and hunger for air. The most interesting and perhaps apt description of dyspnea was given by Jesse, 5 years old and already a testimonial for the American Asthma Association, who said "I feel like a fish out of water."

The severity of this symptom, the speed of its onset and its progression supply us with important information regarding the patient's capacity to tolerate completely spontaneous ventilation, but do not give us any information on the real state of the blood gases, acidosis, and tolerance of and need for ventilation treatment.

Dyspnea is an extremely variable symptom, related to a series of completely different pathogenic mechanisms and it should not, therefore, be a surprise that there is not a clear correlation between the symptom and the severity of the acute respiratory failure. Paradoxically, for the same impairment of respiratory function, a patient who accepts chronically high levels of $PaCO_2$ reports less dyspnea than a patient who battles fiercely to maintain a normal level of carbon dioxide.

The same can be said for patients who undergo repeated asthma attacks, as if the habit of bronchial obstruction could interact in some way with the acute sensation of lack of breath. For this reason the severity of the dyspnea is usually less during an episode of acute-on-chronic respiratory failure.

There are two mechanisms responsible for this phenomenon. The first is related to compensatory retention of bicarbonates, which reduces the acidosis and, therefore, also the minute ventilation. Since the minute ventilation is not increased, the respiratory muscles, which are often compromised from a mechanical point of view in patients with chronic lung disease, are spared additional work. The second mechanism appears to be connected to the endogenous production of endorphins in response to the increased respiratory load; these would reduce the drive increasing the production of CO_2 but maintaining respiratory work at acceptable levels.

Dyspnea can be measured using a scale that is very well known to pulmonologists and is easy to use and understand. Let's measure it then! For example, a score of 3–4 on Borg's scale is already suggestive of an alarming respiratory distress, and documented variations in response to treatment, such as NIV, are equally important. How sad it is, therefore, to see temperature charts in respiratory wards without any trace of information regarding dyspnea or even the respiratory rate.

5.4   Cyanosis, Tachypnea, and Recruitment of Accessory Muscles

The other clinical signs of respiratory distress severe enough to necessitate the use of ventilation treatment are equally variable and nonspecific and, above all, are related to the underlying disorder.

For example, cyanosis, which is the clinical marker of hypoxemia, depends on there being at least 5 g/dL of non-oxygenated hemoglobin in the capillary blood.

In the case of anemia (Hb < 10 g/dL), the degree of hypoxemia must be severe ($SaO_2 = 50$–60 %) before cyanosis is manifested, whereas in a polycythemic patient cyanosis is evident at much higher levels of oxygen in the blood ($SaO_2 > 70$ %).

Tachypnea is a phenomenon often associated with dyspnea and occurs in cases of both respiratory pump failure and parenchymal failure. In patients with COPD, tachypnea is the initial mechanism to compensate for the increased elastic load. The respiratory pattern that these patients adopt is characterized by so-called "rapid, shallow breathing" which, by reducing the inspiratory effort of each breath and, consequently the tidal volume, tends to minimize the total work of the respiratory system as well.

The observation of thoraco-abdominal movements and the use of respiratory muscles, particularly the accessory respiratory muscles, supplies us with an empirical picture of the stage of respiratory distress. The reader is referred to the chapter on monitoring for a detailed analysis of these signs.

5.5   Neurological Status

The neurological status is equally important for deciding whether to start ventilation therapy. Besides the classic Glasgow Coma Scale, which has in any case been found to be relatively insensitive in patients with acute respiratory failure, there are other types of neurological assessments, of which Kelly's scale is the most important, designed to determine the degree of impairment of consciousness in patients with respiratory disorders (Table 5.2). A state of stupor, in which the patient only responds to simple verbal commands or painful stimuli, is definitely a precise indication for ventilation therapy. However, a comatose patient does not necessarily have to be intubated, since there is now evidence in the literature that these patients too can be treated with NIV.

The case is different in very agitated and intolerant patients with a high degree of excitability, which is often an insurmountable barrier to starting NIV unless sedation is used, as will be described in the following chapters.

5.6   Cough Efficacy

The efficacy of the cough reflex should always be evaluated in patients with chronic respiratory disorders. Abundant secretions together with difficulty in expectorating (due to central inhibition of cough or weakness of the expiratory muscles) are relative contraindications to NIV and for this reason in such cases it is preferable to use tracheal intubation, unless recourse is made of traditional techniques (e.g., cough assistance) or alternative ones (e.g., in-exsufflator®, percussionaire®). A surrogate indicator of the capacity to remove secretions is peak

Table 5.2 Kelly's scale

1. Alert. Follows complex 3-step commands
2. Alert. Follows simple commands
3. Lethargic, but arousable. Follows simple commands
4. Stuporous. Patient only intermittently follows simple commands even with vigorous attempts at arousal
5. Comatose with brainstem intact
6. Comatose with brainstem dysfunction

expiratory flow. This can be monitored, for example, in patients with neuromuscular disorders as an indicator of the cough efficacy.

5.7   Other Clinical Considerations

The degree of cardiovascular instability is another parameter to bear in mind when a patient needs to be ventilated. Cardiovascular failure has multiple causes and various clinical signs, of which the most important is a decreased cardiac output, often accompanied by disorders of rhythm and conduction and unstable blood pressure. All these events can be worsened by marked hypoxemia or by an increased workload on the respiratory system through a set of cardiopulmonary reflexes. In these cases, there is a tendency to use invasive ventilation, above all for reasons of safety. Indeed, according to some authorities, NIV is contraindicated in the presence of cardiovascular instability, although there are no studies clearly demonstrating the dangers related to this type of ventilation.

In our opinion, the most important ethical and medical problem is not so much when to start ventilation therapy (particularly invasive ventilation), but rather whether such therapy should be started at all, with the risk of imposing futile treatment.

Faced with a patient with chronic neuromuscular, or pulmonary disease with recurrent episodes of acute respiratory failure there is the serious dilemma of whether to leave the disease to run its natural course or to intervene with extreme therapeutic measures. The percentage of failure of weaning from mechanical ventilation is high in this subgroup of patients and they, therefore, have a high probability of remaining ventilator-dependent.

Besides the fact that we are personally very skeptical about the real improvement in the quality of life of these patients once they have started continuous ventilation therapy via a tracheostomy, there is the major problem of their management by healthcare staff and the compliance of the patient's family who almost always have to make up for the inefficiencies of public services or stand in for them completely. Indeed, it is known that the treatment and care of these patients is almost always entrusted to their relatives and to the voluntary sector, which is still underdeveloped in some countries.

Many other laboratory examinations and diagnostic investigations can help the doctor to refine the diagnosis and make a more precise evaluation of the severity of the patient's condition and thus make the best informed decision on whether, and if so, when to start ventilation therapy. However, the doctor often finds himself alone, in a stressful situation, with little time and perhaps with limited instruments, having to decide the best therapeutic approach. In this regard, we quote a phrase written 40 years ago by Dr. Feinstein, when financial constraints were perhaps not yet such a pressing problem: "If a doctor indiscriminately orders too many tests and investigations, he wastes time, effort and money. Their cost can weigh too heavily on hospital economies; furthermore, an excessive amount of tests may exceed the capacity of a laboratory to produce correct results. If, on the other hand, the doctor orders only a few tests, relying exclusively on his presumed 'clinical eye', without needing objective confirmation, he runs the risk of making serious diagnostic and therapeutic errors."

Suggested Reading

Elliott M, Moxham J (1994) Noninvasive mechanical ventilation by nasal or face mask. In: Tobin M (ed) Principles and practice of mechanical ventilation. McGraw-Hill, New York

Kelly BJ, Matthay MA (1993) Prevalence and severity of neurological dysfunction in critically ill patients. Influence on need for continued mechanical ventilation. Chest 104:1818–1824

Nava S, Hill N (2009) Non-invasive ventilation in acute respiratory failure. Lancet 209(374): 250–259

Nava S, Navalesi P, Conti G (2006) Time of non-invasive ventilation. Intensive Care Med 32(3):361–370

Sancho J, Servera E, Dìaz J, Marìn J (2007) Predictors of ineffective cough during a chest infection in patients with stable amyotrophic lateral sclerosis. Am J Respir Crit Care Med 175(12):1266–1271

How I Ventilate a Patient Non Invasively

6

What is the method of choice for ventilating a patient non invasively? This is one of the most commonly asked questions and yet no one is able to answer since no comparative studies have been published except for a few physiological studies which did not show statistically significant differences between the techniques, except better patient-ventilator synchrony in a few cases. Certainly it is easier to state that the pressure modes (i.e., pressure support and pressure controlled) are much more widely used in clinical practice. Table 6.1 shows estimated percentages of use of the various different modes during episodes of acute respiratory failure, based on published studies.

In this chapter, we describe the main characteristics of the most important types of ventilation, recalling that only the assisted modes (i.e., modes in which the patient can trigger the ventilator) are discussed, since NIV, by definition, can only be applied in patients who have a minimum of respiratory autonomy. There is a lot of confusion between the various abbreviations used for the different modes because, for problems of copyright, the same type of ventilation is named differently depending on the ventilator. For example, proportional-assisted ventilation (PAV) is called that with some ventilators, but by other names with other machines. Another term that creates considerable confusion is BiPAP®, which written in this way is the name of a ventilator, but which has now become synonymous with bilevel ventilation. Furthermore, this acronym should not be confused for BiPAP®, a mode that we shall describe later, developed and available under this name with *Draeger* ventilators. So much for wanting to keep things simple…

6.1 Continuous Positive Airway Pressure

It may surprise some readers, but we have not included CPAP under the section of ventilation modes (see below). This is because it is not actually a true method of ventilation.

S. Nava and F. Fanfulla, *Non Invasive Artificial Ventilation*,
DOI: 10.1007/978-88-470-5526-1_6, © Springer-Verlag Italia 2014

Table 6.1 Estimated percentage use of different modes of NIV during acute respiratory failure	• Pressure support	54 %
	• Pressure controlled	14 %
	• Volume assisted	4 %
	• Proportional assisted	3 %
	• CPAP	23 %
	• Others	2 %

CPAP is, in fact, spontaneous breathing in which ventilation is entrusted entirely to the patient, while the ventilator or pressure generator has the task of maintaining a pre-set positive pressure, i.e., higher than atmospheric pressure, constant for the whole of inspiration (Fig. 6.1). During CPAP, no inspiratory aid is delivered at a positive pressure and for this reason it is incorrect to define CPAP as ventilatory support, according to the previously described equation of motion.

The operator must simply regulate the established level of pressure and the sensitivity of the ventilator, which varies depending on the system used (continuous or on-demand flow). CPAP is often confused in common language with extrinsic PEEP.

The former, as its name indicates, is continuous delivery of pressure, while the latter is involved only in the expiratory phase during some other methods of positive pressure ventilation, such as volume assisted/controlled (A/C) ventilation or pressure support ventilation (PSV), pressure controlled ventilation (PCV), or proportional assist ventilation (PAV).

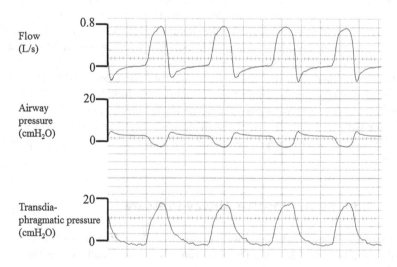

Fig. 6.1 Patient ventilated with CPAP

6.1.1 Applications

Since it is a totally spontaneous mode, it is clear that the CPAP must only be applied in patients with an intact respiratory drive whose respiratory muscles function well. The physiological alterations induced by CPAP, and, therefore, its indications, differ according to the underlying pathology.

In patients with COPD with hypercapnic acute respiratory failure, CPAP can offset the negative effect of the intrinsic PEEP (PEEPi), which we recall contributes substantially (by even more than 60 %) to the work of the inspiratory muscles, during an episode of acute respiratory failure. In any case, great care must be given to the value set, since this must not exceed that of the PEEPi, in order to avoid further hyperinflation in subjects who are already working with increased lung volumes. This entails a reduction in the maximal force of the respiratory muscles which then have to work in a still more unfavorable part of the length/tension curve and an increase in the threshold load that the patient has to overcome before starting a breath. Remember that the dynamic PEEPi recorded in these patients with acute respiratory failure rarely exceeds the threshold of 6–8 cmH$_2$O, while we sometimes see patients with COPD who are being ventilated with levels of CPAP over 10 cmH$_2$O. This is probably because it is impossible to monitor the value of PEEPi adequately, except by measuring transdiaphragmatic pressure (Pdi), as illustrated in Fig. 6.2. This figure shows clearly that the PEEPi is defined as the part of the transdiaphragmatic pressure expended "uselessly" before the flow returns to normal, i.e., to the value at which the respiratory system is in an equilibrium.

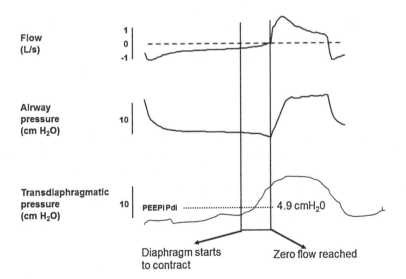

Fig. 6.2 Recognition of intrinsic PEEP

CPAP is still sometimes used in intensive care units in attempts to wean patients with COPD from mechanical ventilation, but the risk of hyperinflation with this level of pressure must never be underestimated.

To our knowledge, there is only one published study on the use of CPAP in hypercapnic acute respiratory failure and we do not, therefore, feel that we can suggest its use in this pathology, except perhaps in association with inspiratory support.

The most rational use of CPAP is in those disorders characterized by nonhypercapnic acute respiratory failure, above all in cases of acute cardiogenic pulmonary edema, but also in cases of thoracic trauma complicated by rib fractures, burns, and in the treatment or prevention of atelectasis. The mechanism through which CPAP improves the state of oxygenation in these conditions is related to the effect that the positive pressure has in contributing to improving lung compliance ("keeping the alveoli open"). In the case of acute cardiogenic pulmonary edema, the hemodynamic effect is equally important and is discussed in detail in the chapter dedicated to the use of NIV in this disorder.

There are three systems through which CPAP can be delivered. The first is the so-called CPAP circuit, or continuous flow system, which includes a series of components (gas blender, reservoir, humidifier, and PEEP valve) through which fresh gases pass at a flow rate of about 30 L/m. This apparatus has the advantage of being inexpensive, easily constructed, and can be assembled by hand. The other two systems of administering CPAP depend on the characteristics of the ventilator.

Some of the old ventilators had an on-demand system (*demand flow*), whereas the more recent ones use a continuous flow system called, depending on the manufacturer, *flow-by* or *bias-flow*. The advantage of this latter system is that it reduces the work of the inspiratory muscles considerably and is widely used when CPAP is delivered via a traditional ventilator, particularly during trials of spontaneous breathing in patients intubated with a T tube. In practice, as far as regards the use of CPAP in NIV, the *stand-alone system*, that is, separate from the ventilator, is definitely the most widely employed, because of its ease of use.

6.2   Volume Modes

A simple rule for understanding how a ventilator mode works is to ask yourself what is/are the variable/s determined by the operator (independent variable/s) and what are their consequences (dependent variable/s). In the final analysis, the person who determines the dependent variables is the patient, through involuntary mechanisms (the mechanical properties of the respiratory system) or voluntary ones (respiratory drive, respiratory rate, etc.).

6.2.1 Assisted/Controlled Ventilation

6.2.1.1 Independent and Dependent Variables During A/C Ventilation

During A/C ventilation, the independent variables (Fig. 6.3) are, logically, the tidal volume set by the operator, the sensitivity of the inspiratory trigger (when this setting is possible) and the time in which this volume is delivered, expressed as the inspiratory time (Ti) or, in some ventilators, as flow.

Remember that the volume is nothing other than the integration of the flow; thus, for a set tidal flow, the velocity of the flow determines the Ti and vice versa. The dependent variables are the airway pressure and respiratory rate.

6.2.1.2 Applications

This is the oldest mode of ventilation but, as mentioned earlier, is now not often used for NIV. It is still popular in North America and countries with a similar school of thought (Australia, South Africa, India, and Central-Southern America) in patients ventilated invasively, while in Europe PSV, PCV, or BiPAP are currently used after the first few days of ventilation even in patients with acute respiratory distress syndrome.

A/C ventilation is a so-called volume-related mode of ventilation. As implicitly indicated from its abbreviation, it can be totally controlled when the sensitivity of the trigger is cancelled and the patient cannot interact with the ventilator, or assisted.

In some ventilators, the two modes are separate and are denoted by the abbreviations CMV and AMV (for controlled mechanical ventilation and assisted mechanical ventilation, respectively), while in most cases they are grouped as a single mode under the abbreviation ACV or A/C with the possibility of excluding or not the trigger.

In the case of "pure" controlled ventilation, most patients also need sedation or even neuromuscular blockade to obtain greater adaptation to this mode, which is typically used only in the first hours of ventilation in severely hypoxic patients.

During assisted ventilation, the sensitivity of the trigger is determined by the operator and the patient is able, having overcome the threshold value with an inspiratory effort, to activate the ventilator. In any case, a minimum frequency is set in order to allow effective ventilation if the patient does not start to take a breath in a period of time that depends on the respiratory rate which has been set. For example, if a minimum respiratory rate of 10 breaths/min is set, every full

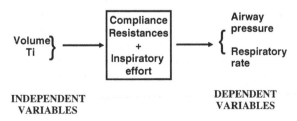

Fig. 6.3 Volume assisted ventilation

breath is quantified as taking 6 s (60/10); if, after this period, the ventilator is not triggered, it automatically starts inflation at a constant volume. Too high a back-up frequency can cause alkalosis, inhibit the patient's respiratory drive or, in the case of a patient with COPD, induce dynamic hyperinflation. There are no apparent advantages of volume A/C ventilation during NIV compared to the more classical pressure methods, since physiological studies have disproven a commonplace belief that the work of respiratory muscles is reduced more during A/C than during other modes of ventilation such as pressure support. It is, therefore, an error to think that volume A/C is the mode of ventilation that minimizes the effort of inspiratory muscles.

The major disadvantages of A/C ventilation include its hemodynamic effects. The cardiac output depends predominantly on venous return, which is determined by the pressure gradient between the right atrium and the systemic venous pressure. Volume-targeted ventilation causes an increase in intrathoracic pressure during inspiration, with a consequent increase in right atrial pressure and decrease in venous return.

One field in which A/C ventilation is still very popular is home ventilation of the patient who cannot be weaned and is, therefore, being ventilated through a tracheotomy tube.

6.2.2 Synchronized Intermittent Mandatory Ventilation

Intermittent mandatory ventilation (IMV) or SIMV is a mode of ventilation that was already studied in the 1950s and that had some success until the 1980s when it was more or less abandoned in clinical practice in many European countries, although remaining very popular in North America and other non-European countries. There are no studies on the use of SIMV during NIV. SIMV was a ventilatory mode originally proposed for the ventilatory treatment of neonates and was used later for weaning post-operative patients and others in whom weaning was difficult.

6.2.2.1 Independent and Dependent Variables During SIMV

Some mandatory breaths, which are set in volume or pressure support or controlled ventilation, are established by the operator (independent variables). Thus, some dependent variables are derived from the type of SIMV used (pressure or volume), as is the timing of these breaths. During the nonassisted breaths, it is the patient who determines his respiratory pattern. In practice, SIMV is a ventilatory support in which a series of breaths are supplied obligatorily with a volume- or pressure-targeted mode by the ventilator but, between one breath and another, the patient can breathe without any support or with a set level of CPAP. In this way, the patient can autonomously vary his breathing pattern and if the mandatory rate is relatively low, the patient may also be able to regain total control of the ventilation. In contrast, when the respiratory rate set by the operator is high, the patient's spontaneous activity is, in practice, suppressed. Between these two extremes there are, of course, ample possibilities for partial support.

6.2.2.2 Applications
SIMV is definitely more advantageous than controlled ventilation. In particular, the patient-ventilator coordination is better since all the patient's inspiratory efforts are picked up by the machine; furthermore, some studies have shown that the risk of barotrauma or volume trauma and the reduction of cardiac output related to high inflation pressures are decreased during SIMV, since the mandatory breaths are interspersed by spontaneous breaths and the mean pressure over a given period of time is lower. Furthermore, SIMV seems to reduce the risk of respiratory alkalosis, improve the distribution of gas within the lungs and prevent disuse atrophy.

The advantages of SIMV with respect to assisted modes of ventilation are less clear.

As far as concerns the comparison with volume-assisted ventilation, the few studies that have been published do not document substantial differences between the two modes with regard to cardiac output, oxygen consumption, and the prevention of respiratory alkalosis. There are no comparative studies of SIMV and PSV during episodes of acute respiratory failure, while a trial in post-operative patients showed that the peak pressure in the airways was lower during PSV. Considering the most common use of SIMV, that is, weaning from mechanical ventilation, it appears to be clearly inferior to both PSV and a trial with a T-tube.

With regard to NIV, many volume-regulated home ventilators include the SIMV option, but to our knowledge this method has never been applied non invasively.

6.3   Pressure Modes

6.3.1   Pressure Support Ventilation

The advent of portable pressure ventilators for NIV, e.g., bilevel ventilators, has increased the enthusiasm for this mode of ventilation and also made it popular among pulmonologists. The clinical advantages of PSV are clear even to the uninitiated, given its good adaptability to the needs of the patient who tolerates it well, both in the early stages of ventilation and during weaning. It is, however, often overlooked that this type of ventilation can have some limitations.

6.3.1.1 Independent and Dependent Variables During PSV
Here we pick up the concept of dependent and independent variables again. During PSV, the independent variables (Fig. 6.4), that is, those set by the operator, are the inspiratory pressure and possibly the expiratory pressure, the threshold of the inspiratory trigger and possibly that of the trigger that controls the cycling between

Fig. 6.4 Flow-cycled
pressure support ventilation

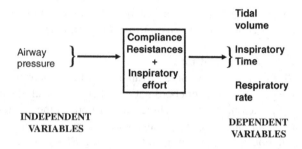

inspiration and expiration. The dependent variables are the inspiratory time, expiratory time, tidal volume, and respiratory rate.

PSV is, therefore, a method of ventilation in which every one of the patient's spontaneous breaths receives an inspiratory pressure support. The inspiratory pressure of the airways is maintained constant at the level established by the operator and since the passage to the expiratory phase is regulated by a drop in flow, the patient should theoretically have complete control of the respiratory timing and tidal volume. This should, at least in theory, improve not only tolerance of the ventilation, but also the interaction between the patient and the machine. Given its characteristics, in some ventilators the PSV mode is, improperly, called "Spontaneous Breathing."

6.3.1.2 Applications

PSV is the most frequently used mode during NIV, perhaps because it is erroneously thought to be the easiest and quickest to set.

From a clinical point of view, the change from any other mode of ventilation to PSV is usually associated with greater comfort and better compliance by the patient. This has been demonstrated in numerous studies, although these have been limited to the acute effect and have not gone further into the longer term effects.

The other major advantage of PSV is that the work of the inspiratory muscles can be graded and personalized according to individual needs by varying the level of pressure support. The addition of extrinsic PEEP or CPAP during PSV can further reduce the work of the respiratory muscles, both during an episode of acute respiratory failure in patients with marked dynamic hyperinflation and during periods of clinical stability. The success of non invasively applied PSV may also be related to the fact that with almost all the most popular so-called home pressure ventilators, an expiratory pressure can also be set (i.e., extrinsic PEEP or CPAP), whereas this is not always possible with home volume ventilators.

As we know, neuromuscular blockade or heavy sedation cannot be used in patients being ventilated non invasively and it is, therefore, important that these patients have a very comfortable and physiological ventilatory support. The field of clinical applications of PSV during NIV is so broad that there are in fact no limitations to its use in either hypoxic or hypercapnic acute respiratory failure. It is, however, clear that in the case of decreased respiratory drive or alterations in breathing during sleep, a back-up frequency, or a switch to a controlled pressure, could be advisable. Having said this, setting all the independent variables correctly is the key to the success of PSV which, as we shall see in the chapter on this subject, is not always as simple as *"I only have to turn a few knobs"*.

In line with this, in some cases, PSV can cause major problems of patient-ventilator interaction. For example, asynchrony between the ventilatory demand of the patient and the response of the ventilator during PSV has now been extensively described in patients with COPD, especially, but not only, if they have considerable emphysema. In particular, it has been demonstrated that numerous ineffective efforts can be made, or the double trigger phenomenon may occur. Intubated patients who develop these anomalous interactions are those who have greater problems with being weaned from ventilation and in whom tracheotomy is more often required. How much the presence of asynchronies affects patients' clinical outcome, in terms of survival, has not yet been studied.

As far as concerns, the hemodynamic effects of this mode of ventilation in patients who are or who are not intubated, minor alterations in the major cardiovascular parameters have been described using a range of pressures. Higher inspiratory pressures (~ 30 cmH$_2$O) and respiratory rate (20 breaths/min) were recently adopted to ventilate chronic hypercapnic COPD patients in order to achieve the maximal PaCO$_2$ reduction. This type of approach called high-intensity positive pressure mechanical ventilation (Hi-NPPV), has been shown to improve spontaneous diurnal blood gases better than the traditional lower pressures approach (Li-NPPV). It was, however, found in a later physiological study, that a significant reduction of cardiac output was present, when a total reduction of inspiratory effort, with an increased in intrathoracic pressure was achieved.

6.3.2 Pressure Controlled Ventilation

PCV is a mode of pressure ventilation which approaches, with due differences, the volume A/C mode. Its underlying principle, like that of PSV, is to supply a pressure support in which the cycling between inspiration is not caused by a decrease in flow and, therefore, in the final analysis, by the respiratory mechanics of the patient but are pre-set by the operator.

The most widely used form of PCV during NIV is time-cycled and it is this that we discuss below.

6.3.2.1 Independent and Dependent Variables During PCV

During PCV, the independent variables (Fig. 6.5), that is, the variables set by the operator, are inspiratory pressure and possibly also expiratory pressure, the threshold of the inspiratory trigger and the inspiratory time for which this pressure is maintained.

As for the volume-controlled modality, there are ventilators with which the patient cannot interact and so a trigger cannot be set. The dependent variables are

Fig. 6.5 Time-cycled pressure controlled ventilation

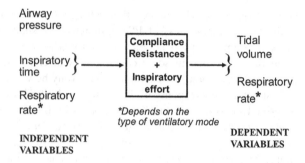

the tidal volume and the respiratory rate, this latter only in the case that the ventilator allows triggering.

Once the parameters have been specified, the mean pressure in the airways and, therefore, also approximately the alveolar pressure, should not exceed a given established value, but as for PSV the Vt, the minute ventilation and the alveolar ventilation cannot be controlled since these vary depending on the changes in respiratory mechanics.

6.3.2.2 Applications

The advantage of PCV is that it can be applied in patients who have reduced respiratory drive or marked muscle weakness, contemporaneously reducing the risk of volume trauma or barotrauma, compared with that of volume-controlled ventilation, in the case that respiratory mechanics change unexpectedly. PCV is also used in cases of air leaks, when the ventilators used (particularly old generation intensive care ones) are not able to compensate for the air-leaks. In fact in the case of PSV the cycling threshold between inspiration and expiration could be reached only after an unacceptably long period of time if, because of the air losses, the flow does not decrease to values pre-established by the ventilator's algorithm. This phenomenon, which is increasingly rare with modern ventilators, is called *hang-up*; the term indicates the patient's inability to finish the inspiratory phase while the machine continues to insufflate air.

6.3.3   Proportional Assist Ventilation

This is definitely a very interesting method of ventilation, although honestly it is little used in clinical practice. Why? The first reason is that not all ventilators allow this option, which is not currently registered in the USA since it has not yet been approved by the Food and Drug Administration; secondly, given that it is based on not immediately comprehensible physiological concepts, it is often viewed with suspicion by clinicians.

As shown in Fig. 6.6, unlike PSV, in which the pressure support during inspiration is pre-determined, PAV provides a sort of support proportional to the

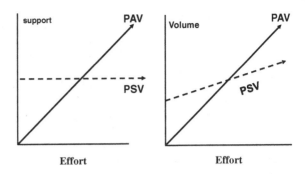

Fig. 6.6 Difference between PAV and PSV

patient's effort. Theoretically, this mode should allow automatic synchrony with changes in the patient's ventilatory demand.

6.3.3.1 Independent and Dependent Variables During PAV

PAV and PSV have some basic characteristics in common, in particular the fact that both modes were designed to support spontaneous inspiratory efforts by supplying a certain level of pressure support to the airways. It is difficult to establish the independent and dependent variables in this mode. In fact, with PAV no airway pressure, flow or tidal volume is set *a priori*; instead, the aim is to guarantee instant by instant a support in relation to the patient's effort.

During assisted ventilation, the pressure applied to the respiratory system (Prs) is given by the pressure of the respiratory muscles (Pmus) and by the ventilator (Paw), which represents the level of "external" assistance to the patient. Thus:

$$P_{rs} = P_{mus} + P_{aw}$$

All of us, and patients in particular, must overcome an elastic load and a resistive load and so the patient's effort can be determined by the formula:

$$P_{mus} = R \times V + E \times VT + PEEPi - P_{aw}$$

where V is the flow, VT is the volume generated, R is the resistance, E is the elastance and PEEPi is the instrinsic PEEP.

In PAV, during the inspiratory phase, the ventilator generates a positive pressure proportional to the flow and volume generated by the patient and, therefore:

$$P_{aw} = FA \times V + VA \times VT$$

Consequently, the more force the patient generates, the more the machine assists him and vice versa.

The operator can set the level of assistance of flow and volume, in this way "modulating" the effort of the patient with respect to his conditions.

Thus, from a practical point of view, only a single parameter needs to be regulated in PAV, that is, the percentage of the patient's *compliance* and resistance that the ventilator must be responsible for. Assuming that the measurements of respiratory mechanics are correct, setting the assistance to 100 % would reduce the patient's respiratory work to a minimum, whereas setting it at zero would maximize the patient's work.

What becomes critical when setting the ventilatory assistance is the measurement of the *compliance* and resistances (those of the endotracheal tube are subtracted). The most scientific method would be to measure these parameters during the brief period of controlled volume ventilation, but if this is not possible, there are two alternatives during PAV.

The first is based on the method of occluding the airways during an inspiration maintained for the whole expiratory cycle. The elastance or *compliance* (its reciprocal) is calculated using mathematical formulae.

The second, more empirical, but practical method for measuring elastance and, thereby choosing the level of respiratory assistance, is the so-called "*runaway*".

The operator gradually increases the degree of volume assist until the level at which the ventilator can no longer cycle the breath in the usual time and so the inspiratory time becomes prolonged for a long period. This value of volume assist is usually just greater than the patient's elastance and so this latter can be determined without requiring particular equations.

The new PAV*plus* option is able to monitor the resistance and elastance values automatically and, therefore, considerably simplifies setting the ventilator.

6.3.3.2 Applications

There are now both physiological and clinical studies that have been able to demonstrate the clinical efficacy of PAV in chronic and acute respiratory failure, and in this latter case in both hypercapnic and hypoxemic forms. Most of the research has focused on the comparison with PSV, showing the "noninferiority" of PAV with respect to the more consolidated method. Furthermore, PAV seems to be better tolerated, at least in the first hours of ventilation, induces better patient-ventilator synchrony and also improves the quality of sleep in the intensive care unit. The new PAV*plus* seems to offer further improvements compared to traditional PAV, by automatically monitoring respiratory mechanics at predetermined intervals and thereby enabling changes of the settings of the flow and volume assists "in course". However, as said earlier, the presumed easier use of PSV limits the use of PAV in clinical practice. But we also know how difficult it is in medicine to change the ideas and, even more so, the habits of someone who has used a method for years and which has, in any case given satisfaction.

Suggested Reading

Appendini L, Patessio A, Zanaboni S (1994) Physiologic effects of positive end-expiratory pressure and mask pressure support during exacerbations of chronic obstructive pulmonary disease. Am J Respir Crit Care Med 149(5):1069–1076

Brochard L (2002) Intrinsic (or auto) PEEP during controlled mechanical ventilation. Intensive Care Med 28(1):1376–1378

Brochard L, Pluskwa F, Lemaire F (1987) Improved efficacy of spontaneous breathing with inspiratory pressure support. Am Rev Respir Dis 136(2):411–415

Dreher M, Storre JH, Schmoor C et al (2010) High-intensity versus low-intensity non-invasive ventilation in patients with stable hypercapnic COPD: a randomised crossover trial. Thorax 65:303–308

Gay PC, Hess DR, Hill NS (2001) Noninvasive proportional assist ventilation for acute respiratory insufficiency. Comparison with pressure support ventilation. Am J Respir Crit Care Med 164(9):106–111

Lukácsovits J, Carlucci A, Hill N, Ceriana P, Pisani L, Schreiber A, Pierucci P, Losonczy G, Nava S (2012) Physiological changes during low and high "intensity" noninvasive ventilation. Eur Respir J 39:869–875

MacIntyre NR, Ho LI (1991) Effects of initial flow rate and breath termination criteria on pressure support ventilation. Chest 99(1):134–138

Nava S, Ambrosino N, Rubini F (1993) Effect of nasal pressure support ventilation and external PEEP on diaphragmatic activity in patients with severe stable COPD. Chest 103(1):143–150

Nava S, Bruschi C, Rubini F (1995) Respiratory response and inspiratory effort during pressure support ventilation in COPD patients. Intensive Care Med 21(11):871–879

Petrof BJ, Legaré M, Goldberg P (1990) Continuous positive airway pressure reduces work of breathing and dyspnea during weaning from mechanical ventilation in severe chronic obstructive pulmonary disease. Am Rev Respir Dis 141(2):281–829

Sassoon C, Zhu E, Caiozzo VJ (2004) Assist-control mechanical ventilation attenuates ventilator-induced diaphragmatic dysfunction. Am J Respir Crit Care Med 170(6):626–632

How I Set a Ventilator

7

Setting a ventilator is only apparently easy and requires some notions of respiratory physiology, because the setting of some parameters can directly influence others.

Before doing anything to the ventilator and, therefore, to the patient, always ask yourself the simple questions: what are the independent variables, what are the dependent ones, and how much can the patient's conditions influence these latter? For example, is it worth starting Pressure Support ventilation with values higher than 20 cmH$_2$O in an emphysematous patient, that is, a patient with a high compliance, in whom we could perhaps obtain a suitable tidal volume at lower pressures?

7.1 What do Volume and Pressure Mode Settings Have in Common?

7.1.1 The Trigger

During assisted mode ventilation, the breath supplied by the ventilator is a response to the patient's inspiratory effort. The effort required by the patient to start a cycle is decided by the operator who sets the level of sensitivity of the trigger.

There are various types of trigger, but the main ones are pressure and flow. Neither of these is instantaneous and there is a certain delay between the beginning of the inspiratory effort and the start of the ventilator. The way these triggers work is illustrated schematically in Fig. 7.1. Some ventilators specifically dedicated to NIV also use so-called mixed triggers in which the algorithm recognizes more than one triggering mechanism from among pressure, flow, and volume on the basis of the concept that "whichever of the three reaches the criteria set first, activates the trigger." Unfortunately, most companies do not release more precise information on these algorithms, particularly when the triggering system is automatic and not, therefore, modifiable by the operator.

S. Nava and F. Fanfulla, *Non Invasive Artificial Ventilation*,
DOI: 10.1007/978-88-470-5526-1_7, © Springer-Verlag Italia 2014

Fig. 7.1 a "Classical" flow or pressure trigger. **b** Flow-by trigger system

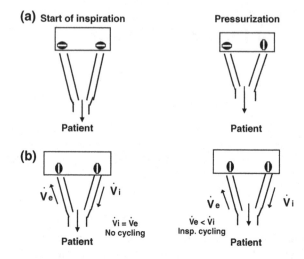

As far as concerns a pressure trigger, this is usually set by the operator at around -1 cmH$_2$O. In some types of ventilator, the minimum sensitivity is 0.3 cmH$_2$O, while others start directly from 1 cmH$_2$O. The maximum sensitivity threshold used in clinical practice almost never exceeds 2–3 cmH$_2$O.

One error not to make is to set a "hard" trigger with the aim of training the respiratory muscles for a possible attempt at weaning from the ventilator. This strategy is a mistake, both physiologically and clinically. In fact, first, the diaphragm and respiratory muscles of the vast majority of patients with chronic respiratory disorders are sufficiently exercised by years of "training" against a natural elastic and resistive load. Second, training respiratory muscles could lead to destruction of the sarcomeres and damage to the muscle fibers themselves. Furthermore, there is no experimental clinical evidence to justify this strategy in ventilated patients.

Excluding cases of extreme muscle weakness, in the case of preserved respiratory drive, the delay in a pressure trigger depends on intrinsic factors such as the microprocessor, the pressure transducer, the circuit, any humidification and, above all, on the system of valves being used (pneumatic or solenoid). An example of delayed triggering is illustrated in Fig. 7.2. The patient starts the effort (the Pdi signal is positive) at the moment that the flow is zero and there is, therefore, no auto-PEEP, but this is not followed in real time by flow and pressure support by the machine, which is activated "only" after 87 ms. Of course, any PEEPi present must be taken into consideration when calculating the trigger delay.

A flow trigger, now supplied with almost all ventilators, seems to enable significant reductions in both the work of the patient's inspiratory muscles and the delay in opening the valves. These systems are based on the so-called flow-by or *bias-flow*, which consists of a continuous supply of a constant flow; variations in the flow, caused by the inspiratory effort, between the inspiratory and expiratory arms are detected by a sensor that determines the start of the mechanical cycle.

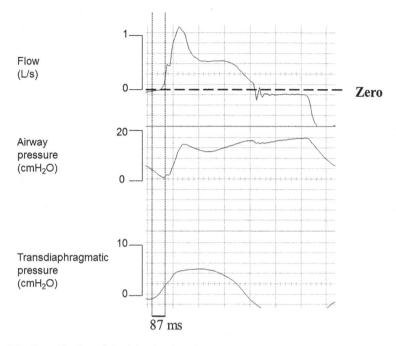

Fig. 7.2 Quantification of the delay in triggering

The threshold of the trigger, equivalent to the delta of the pressure generated by the patient, can vary from 1 to 10 L/m and is usually set at 2–3 L/m. The advantages of this type of trigger, compared to the pressure trigger, are the result of the fact that the constant basal flow artificially produces a sort of external PEEP, which in itself reduces the level of inspiratory effort in patients with auto-PEEP.

In the most extreme cases, the level of the PEEPi is so high that the patient's respiratory effort does not reach the minimum criteria for triggering and the ventilator does not, therefore, supply pressure in response to the patient's inspiration.

When the operator has the possibility of choosing, or even setting, the trigger, our advice is to use a flow trigger with a higher threshold, although without causing self-triggering phenomena at the same time.

Many ventilators for NIV do not allow absolute values to be used to set the trigger; the trigger is set according to a numerical scale of sensitivity, usually from 1 to 5.

7.1.2   The Respiratory Rate

The respiratory rate during volume- and pressure-assisted ventilation is usually set at 10–14 breaths/min. Of course, the setting of the respiratory rate depends on the type of the patient and his characteristics. It is worth monitoring the sleep profile of patients ventilated during the night in order to avoid changes in the patient/respirator synchrony in the presence of, for example, central type apnea. In the controlled modalities, the respiratory rate determines the expiratory time once the flow and the tidal volume have been established. For example, if these latter parameters are maintained stable, an increase in the respiratory rate is associated with a decrease in the expiratory time and vice versa. In recent years, there has been a tendency in North European countries to ventilate patients with stable hypercapnia with a technique called high intensity ventilation, which is characterized by a fast breathing rate (>20 breaths/min) and high inspiratory pressures (values >20–25 cmH$_2$O). In reality, there is little scientific evidence to support this strategy (i.e., no large randomized controlled trials), some potential side effects need to be taken into consideration, such as a reduction in cardiac output and the air losses occurring at these pressures.

7.1.3   Fraction of Inspired Oxygen

The fraction of inspired oxygen (FiO$_2$) is a parameter that is often little considered, particularly during NIV. In the past, pulmonologists (we) were accustomed to ventilate our first patients with ventilators that only allowed the delivery of low flows of oxygen through an external port (i.e., mask, connection introduced into the circuit). This had a certain logic given that until a few years ago the vast majority of patients receiving NIV had COPD which, by definition, does not require a particularly high FiO$_2$ to reach a satisfactory SaO$_2$. However, the expansion of the applications of NIV has led to the problem of having to guarantee a higher concentration of oxygen for some types of patient, such as those with acute pulmonary edema, pneumonia, or acute lung injury (ALI)/acute respiratory distress syndrome (ARDS). All intensive care ventilators and most ventilators designed specifically for NIV are able to supply a FiO$_2$ up to 100 % since they are endowed with a blender.

We would, however, like to go back for a while to the problem of supplementary oxygen in COPD. Our practical advice is to monitor the patient at all times with an oximeter and to regulate the FiO$_2$ to obtain values of SaO$_2$ around 88–92 % in order to avoid worsening the acidosis due to inappropriate administration of a high FiO$_2$. How many cases of severe acidosis have developed in the journey between home and hospital when relatives or, worse still, healthcare staff, have raised the level of oxygen too high in order to "help the patient breathe better"?

7.2 Specific Setting of Volume Modes

7.2.1 Tidal Volume

During volume modes of ventilation, the tidal volume is an INDEPENDENT variable. There has been much discussion on setting the tidal volume and many studies to determine its most appropriate values.

First of all, it is a mistake to think of a setting in absolute terms; it is more appropriate to define a tidal volume based on the weight of the patient. In contrast to prevailing thought until a few years ago and to indeed to what we wrote in the previous edition of this book, values of 6–8 mL/kg should not be exceeded (except on rare occasions) during either invasive or non invasive ventilation. Many studies in patients with ARDS have established that the gold standard A/C ventilation is that at low volumes (<6 mL/kg) which can lead on the one hand to alveolar hypoventilation (or permissive hypercapnia), but on the other hand avoids the effects of volume trauma and, consequently, also the so-called biotrauma due to alveolar distress with the release of mediators of inflammation.

This strategy has improved the survival of patients with ARDS, reducing the above-described, known complications.

As far as concerns more specifically pneumological patients, that is, patients with COPD, it makes sense to deliver sufficient volumes to improve the alveolar hypoventilation (i.e., to reduce the $PaCO_2$) without, however, decreasing the $PaCO_2$ level too much. We should remember that these patients live in a stable condition of hypercapnia, that is, with levels of carbon dioxide above the normal values, so there is no sense in ventilating them mechanically in order to obtain carbon dioxide values at the lower limit of normal. One practical tip is never to deliver volumes greater than 8 mL/kg. Larger volumes, besides increasing the risk of volume trauma, could facilitate the development of a poor patient/ventilator interaction (see the following chapters).

From a physiological point of view, when choosing a volume or a rate, it is important not to forget the role of the dead space and the alveolar volume.

The minute volume supplied by the ventilator is given by the product of the tidal volume and the respiratory rate, while the alveolar minute volume is given by the product of the alveolar volume and the respiratory rate. With two different settings of the ventilator, it is, therefore, possible to obtain the same minute volume, but markedly different alveolar minute volumes.

For example, a Vt of 0.25 L associated with a breathing frequency of 20 breaths/min and a Vt of 0.5 L with a respiratory rate of 10 breaths/min both generate a minute volume of 5 L.

If, however, we consider a dead space of 0.15 L, in the former case the alveolar minute volume will be 2.0 L, whereas in the latter case it will be 3.5 L.

One particular problem of NIV, in the few cases in which the volume mode is used, is that of airway losses. In fact, working in a half open system, in most cases the tidal volume set by the operator is not that exhaled by the patient.

7.2.2   Expiratory Pressure

We have included this subchapter for each of the main modes of ventilation because in the severely hypoxic patient (i.e., one with ARDS, usually ventilated with a volume mode; acidotic and hypercapnic, usually ventilated with a pressure mode) the setting of the expiratory pressure (CPAP or external PEEP) has different meanings.

In fact, the main aim of the expiratory pressure when using the volume mode is to recruit areas of parenchyma that are inadequately ventilated because of reduced compliance. As far as concerns, the setting of the external positive pressure in this circumstance, we lack a real, "recipe" agreed by everyone.

Recording a compliance curve can certainly help to identify the so-called inflection point, above which the pulmonary compliance regains a normal slope (Fig. 7.3), but it is not clear whether the positive pressure must be regulated precisely on the point or above it. One concept to keep in mind is that of "opening the lungs," with the delivery of a volume, and then "keeping them open," with the application of external PEEP. In any case, there is a tendency to limit the mean pressures in the airways.

7.2.3   Inspiratory Flow

From a physical point of view, the inspiratory flow is the amount of volume that is administered in a given period of time. Thus, for parity of volume delivered, a high flow means a shorter inspiratory time (T_i) and vice versa. This is why the T_i, rather than the flow, is used as the setting parameter in some volume-mode ventilators.

The flow is a determinant of the patient's respiratory work: in fact, if the flow velocity is too low with respect to requirements, the patient will increase his inspiratory effort in an attempt to meet his own needs. In most respirators used in Intensive Care, the shape of the wave form can be chosen from among four possible options:

Fig. 7.3 Compliance or pressure/volume curve

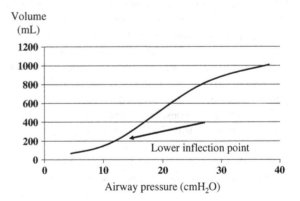

- square wave;
- decelerated flow;
- accelerated flow;
- sinusoidal flow.

Patients without particular lung problems have not been shown to gain benefit from one particular flow wave rather than another. In contrast, in 14 ventilator-dependent patients it was found that the decelerated wave form produced significant improvements in gas exchange and lung mechanics, without altering hemodynamic status. These data were not, however, confirmed by another study carried out in the same population with the same method. We do not, therefore, feel that we can advise any particular type of flow wave.

7.2.4 Inspiratory/Expiratory Ratio

The relationship between inspiratory and expiratory times, or the I:E ratio, is indirectly determined by the setting of other parameters, such as respiratory rate and inspiratory flow. Of course, in patients ventilated with the volume-controlled mode, the I:E ratio is virtually stable at the values set by the operator. During assisted modalities, this ratio varies from breath to breath, depending on the patient's respiratory rate. For example, if I set a breathing rate of 20 breaths/min and an inspiratory time of 1 s, the I:E ratio is 1:3, but if my patient "takes" five supplementary breaths, the ratio will decrease to 1:2.4. The I:E ratio is classically set at 1:2 in patients not affected by chronic lung disorders, whereas in those with COPD, the ratio should be brought to 1:2.5 or 1:3 to enable a longer expiratory time.

7.2.5 Setting Pressure Modes

7.2.5.1 Inspiratory Pressure
During pressure modes of ventilation, inspiratory pressure is an INDEPENDENT variable. Although setting the inspiratory pressure is apparently simple, it is actually full of hazards.

For example, a patient's alveolar ventilation depends on three physiological variables: tidal volume, respiratory rate, and dead space.

If we forget this last variable, which we cannot change, the pressure-assisted modalities will not determine a priori either the tidal volume or the respiratory rate.

This is not the case for the volume modalities, in which at least the tidal volume is determined by the operator. For example, for similar inspiratory pressure (e.g., 15 cmH_2O) and lung resistances, a patient with high compliance (e.g., a patient with emphysema) can develop a tidal volume of 500 mL, while another patient with reduced compliance (e.g., a patient with ARDS) generates much smaller volumes, sometimes even less than 200 mL.

Furthermore, depending on the level of support set by the operator, the patient can receive full assistance for his effort, almost simulating controlled mode ventilation, or, if the inspiratory pressure is lower, the patient can be given only marginal aid.

Unfortunately, the optimal setting of Pressure Support is not as simple as it might seem at first sight and without the help of an esophageal probe, necessary to monitor the pleural pressure, it is not easy, even for expert operators, to establish whether the support offered to the patients is appropriate, underestimated, or overestimated. Certainly we do sometimes see patients, even several days after an acute episode and in a stable condition, being ventilated with Pressure Support that exceeds their real needs. We remind you that almost complete rest of the respiratory muscles can lead to atrophy of these muscles, with consequent difficulty in the process of weaning.

For all the above-listed reasons and despite numerous attempts to define a gold standard for the ventilator setting, no such standard exists, although, in theory, the statements in the chapter on setting volume modalities of ventilation could be valid: that is, pressure support should not generate tidal volumes >8 mL/kg in patients with COPD and >6 mL/kg in those with ARDS. We should, however, remember that at least in the first stages of ventilation, pressure modes are almost never used in ARDS.

Another confounding factor is that related to the definition of inspiratory pressure.

Inspiratory pressure, or Pressure Support, means the real inspiratory aid above the PEEP that is supplied by the ventilator. The term Inspiratory Peak Airways Pressure (IPAP) has a different meaning: it defines the total value of the inspiratory pressure supplied, including the level of PEEP. The vast majority of ventilators for NIV and single-limb ventilators follow this latter logic, while all intensive care ventilators are based on the Pressure Support principle. We hope that Fig. 7.4 resolves this confusion once and for all. In the panel on the left, which refers to an intensive care ventilator, there is a pressure support of 15 cmH$_2$O, which is added to an external PEEP of 5 cmH$_2$O. The total inspiratory pressure that the patient receives is 20 cmH$_2$O, formed of the 5 cmH$_2$O of external PEEP and the 15 cmH$_2$O of Pressure Support. In the panel on the right, which refers to a bilevel ventilator designed for NIV, the IPAP is 15 cmH$_2$O and the external PEEP is 5 cmH$_2$O. In this case, the total pressure is 15 cmH$_2$O, with the patient receiving Pressure Support of 10 cmH$_2$O and an external PEEP of 5 cmH$_2$O.

This "language" problem still creates much confusion. Just consider the case of a patient who is transferred from an ICU to a respiratory ward with a prescription for Pressure Support of 15 cmH$_2$O and an external PEEP of 5 cmH$_2$O. The correct, new setting of a bilevel NIV ventilator should be 20 cmH$_2$O of IPAP and 5 cmH$_2$O of external PEEP.

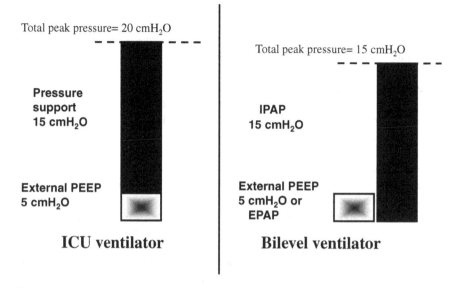

Total peak pressure= 20 cmH$_2$O

Total peak pressure= 15 cmH$_2$O

**Pressure
support
15 cmH$_2$O**

**IPAP
15 cmH$_2$O**

**External PEEP
5 cmH$_2$O**

**External PEEP
5 cmH$_2$O or
EPAP**

ICU ventilator   Bilevel ventilator

Fig. 7.4 The two main algorithms used by different ventilators during pressure support ventilation

7.2.5.2 Expiratory Pressure

The addition of positive expiratory pressure during ventilation with Pressure Support is often called bilevel ventilation, which probably took its name from the first portable ventilators for NIV which were, and still are, called bilevel or Bi-PAP®. Many of these ventilators apply a default continuous flow to facilitate the function of the algorithm that enables compensation for losses. They do, therefore, generate a continuous positive pressure which, depending on the model used, varies from 2 to 4 cmH$_2$O.

As already stated several times, the rationale for the combined use of Pressure Support and CPAP or external PEEP differs between hypercapnic patients and those with "pure" hypoxia.

During exacerbations of COPD, the aim of positive pressure is to reduce the resistive load necessary to eliminate the component of respiratory work due to the presence of intrinsic PEEP. The dynamic hyperinflation characteristic of decompensations in a chronically ill patient causes the values of intrinsic PEEP to rise, reaching values as high as 10 cmH$_2$O or more in some cases. What expiratory pressures should we set in these cases? This is a very common question, but one that is extremely difficult to answer because it is practically impossible to measure the level of intrinsic PEEP directly in clinical practice; this parameter can only be determined by invasive measurements of transdia-phragmatic pressure, which are performed in very few specialized centers. Physiology tells us that the work due to the intrinsic PEEP component accounts for approximately 50 % of the total respiratory work and that to abolish this component almost completely a "counter-PEEP" (i.e., CPAP or external PEEP) of 75–80 % of the intrinsic PEEP is needed (Fig. 7.5). However, physiological studies warn us of the deleterious effects of a CPAP that exceeds the real levels of the intrinsic PEEP, i.e., the risk of further hyperinflation.

Our practical advice is, therefore, to apply always and in any case, a CPAP between 4 and 6 cmH$_2$O in order to reduce the respiratory work without running too high a risk of harming the patient. What if we apply a CPAP of 6 cmH$_2$O and the patient actually has an intrinsic PEEP of 12 cmH$_2$O? We will in any case cancel 50 % of the work due to this component, but it would be very much more serious to set a CPAP of 10 cmH$_2$O in a patient who actually has an intrinsic PEEP of "only" 4 cmH$_2$O, given that in this way we would increase his functional residual capacity (FRC). Since evidence-based medicine does not always help us, as in these cases, we must use a bit of common sense.

The case of a hypoxic patient is very different. As we have already seen, it is better to ventilate a patient with ARDS with volume modes and invasively; having said that, acute pulmonary edema and pneumonia are hypoxic disorders in which it makes sense to use bilevel ventilation. In these cases, setting the external PEEP or CPAP is perhaps easier because it is based on the SaO$_2$ recording. Our advice is to start with low expiratory pressures ($\sim$5 cmH$_2$O) and progressively increase by 1–2 units until reaching a point at which, almost by magic, the SaO$_2$ improves dramatically.

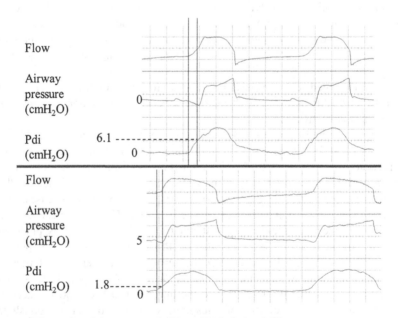

Fig. 7.5 Effects of applying external PEEP or CPAP during PSV

7.2.5.3 Pressurization Phase or Ramp

Once the inspiratory phase has started, the respirator delivers a flow of gas that is modulated during the inspiratory cycle in accordance with the patient's inspiratory effort. The machine's software maintains the flow necessary to reach the pressure predetermined by the operator maintaining it constant until the end of the expiratory phase. With many models of ventilators, the initial flow rate can be varied; a high pressurization rate typically gives a square pressure wave, while a slower one reaches the predetermined pressure level more slowly (Fig. 7.6).

There has been much discussion on the optimal use of this parameter. The faster the ramp time, the less effort the patient makes. This is particularly important in the first stages of ventilation, when the patient has a high drive and is hungry for air. It is of no coincidence that the patient undergoing NIV complains in these phases that "not much air reaches me." The most instinctive behavior would be to increase the inspiratory support, but in fact it might be sufficient to increase the flow rate. It is equally true that, once stabilized, the patient could report that "I'm being given too much air," because the ramp is set too fast. Furthermore, it must be remembered that during NIV an initial inspiratory flow that is too high, or at any rate greater than the patient's requirements, could increase losses and, therefore, decrease the patient's tolerance of the ventilation.

7.2.5.4 Phase of End Inspiration or Start of Expiration

Cycling between the inspiratory/expiratory phases is caused by a drop in the inspiratory flow to a given set value. Usually this threshold value, equivalent to the expiratory trigger, is set by default, although it can also be established by the operator and is expressed as an absolute value or as a fixed percentage of the peak inspiratory flow. Decreased inspiratory flow is the manifestation of the physiological phenomenon that the inspiratory muscles have stopped contracting, but the drop in flow has different characteristics in the various pathologies.

Fig. 7.6 Pressure waves

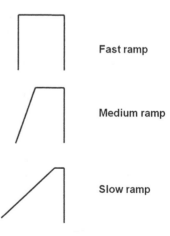

Fast ramp

Medium ramp

Slow ramp

Fig. 7.7 Effect of different
settings of the expiratory
trigger regulated by the drop
of flow during pressure
support ventilation

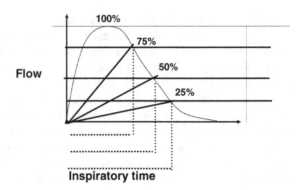

For example, in patients with marked obstruction, the decrease could be too slow and, for this reason, if the expiratory trigger is too "far" from the peak flow, the time to reach the threshold value would be too long. This produces asynchrony phenomena between the patient and the ventilator, although these can be easily corrected given the possibility of raising the threshold. The expiratory trigger obviously directly influences the inspiratory time of the ventilator. For example, as shown in Fig. 7.7, a proposed threshold fall to 75 % of the peak flow is manifested by a very much shorter inspiratory time than that with a higher threshold (e.g., 25 % of the peak flow). During NIV, the possibility of determining the expiratory trigger is particularly useful when there are losses, to which the ventilator reacts by increasing the flow supplied and, thereby, making its rapid decrease more difficult. The safety option that some ventilators have is particularly useful in these cases; this option is a maximum time limit for which inspiration can be maintained, because in the case of losses from the circuit, the cycling mechanism may not function.

7.2.5.5 Inspiratory Time

During Pressure Support ventilation, the T_i can be set in the so-called PCV modality, in which cycling between inspiration and expiration is no longer regulated by the decrease in flow, but by the T_i regulated by the operator. In my opinion, the definition of PCV is inappropriate (in fact, with the vast majority of ventilators the patient is free to trigger the start of inspiration), since the operator is not able to establish the I:E ratio, which could vary from breath to breath. The regulation of the T_i is exclusively dependent on the patient's conditions, although it should be remembered that too short a T_i could generate insufficient tidal volumes whereas too long a T_i could be poorly tolerated by the patient. In order to avoid these potential inconveniences in some ventilators, a range of T_i can be established: below this range the patient cannot activate the expiratory flow trigger and above it the ventilator passes automatically to the expiratory phase.

Suggested Reading

Crotti S, Mascheroni D, Caironi P (2001) Recruitment and derecruitment during acute respiratory failure: a clinical study. Am J Respir Crit Care Med 164(1):131–140

Dreher M, Storre JH, Schmoor C et al (2010) High-intensity versus low-intensity non-invasive ventilation in patients with stable hypercapnic COPD: a randomised crossover trial. Thorax 65:303–308

Laghi F (2003) Effect of inspiratory time and flow settings during assist-control ventilation. Curr Opin Crit Care 9(1):39–44

Lukácsovits J, Carlucci A, Hill N, Ceriana P, Pisani L, Schreiber A, Pierucci P, Losonczy G, Nava S (2012) Physiological changes during low and high "intensity" non-invasive ventilation. Eur Respir J 39:869–875

Nava S, Ambrosino N, Bruschi C (1997) Physiological effects of flow and pressure triggering during non-invasive mechanical ventilation in patients with chronic obstructive pulmonary disease. Thorax 52(3):249–254

Prianianakis G, Delmastro M, Carlucci A et al (2004) Effect of varying the pressurisation rate during non-invasive pressure support ventilation. Eur Respir J 23(2):314–320

Rubenfeld GD, Cooper C, Carter G et al (2004) Barriers to providing lung-protective ventilation to patients with acute lung injury. Crit Care Med 32(6):1289–1293

Stell JM, Paul G, Lee KC (2001) Non-invasive ventilator triggering in chronic obstructive pulmonary disease: a test lung comparison. Am J Respir Crit Care Med 164(11):2092–2097

Tassaux D, Gainnier M, Battisti A, Jolliet P (2005) Impact of expiratory trigger setting on delayed cycling and inspiratory muscle workload. Am J Respir Crit Care Med 172(10): 1283–1289

The Acute Respiratory Distress Syndrome Network (2000) Ventilation with lower tidal volumes as compared with traditional tidal volumes for acute lung injury and the acute respiratory distress syndrome. New Engl J Med 342(18):1301–1308

The Acute Respiratory Distress Syndrome Network (2004) Higher vs lower positive end-expiratory pressures in patients with ARDS. New Engl J Med 351:327–336

Yang SC, Yang SP (2002) Effects of inspiratory flow waveforms on lung mechanics, gas exchange and respiratory metabolism in COPD patients during mechanical ventilation. Chest 122(6):1096–1104

Other Modes of Ventilation

8

Here, we describe very briefly some modes of ventilation that are relatively rarely used, but which theoretically have a rationale for future use in NIV. Many methods that are discreetly popular during invasive mechanical ventilation are, therefore, excluded.

8.1 Neurally Adjusted Ventilatory Assist

Unfortunately, despite the identical name, one of the two authors of this book has nothing to do with neurally adjusted ventilatory assist (NAVA) and will, therefore, never become rich in the case of an explosion of use of this form of ventilation, which remains one of the greatest innovations of recent years.

The functional principle underlying its design is ingenious. As highlighted by Fig. 8.1 all the assisted methods discussed so far are based on the principle that a patient activates the ventilator with a mechanical impulse (i.e., generation of a flow, pressure, or volume), recorded by the ventilator close to the upper airways and, therefore, a long way away from where the impulse to breathe starts (in the central nervous system). Furthermore, there are disorders, such as COPD, characterized by the presence of intrinsic PEEP (PEEPi), which must be overcome in any case to enable activation of the trigger.

Besides the force, the time necessary to overcome the component due to the PEEPi always creates a delay between the contraction of the respiratory muscles and the start of the ventilator support. This can lead to problems of synchrony and poor adaptation. NAVA resolves these problems by measuring the signal for the trigger directly at the level of the diaphragm, recording its electrical activity with an esophageal electrode. Theoretically, therefore, a response from the ventilator should be obtained almost concomitantly with diaphragmatic contraction and, therefore, totally independently of the presence or absence of PEEPi.

S. Nava and F. Fanfulla, *Non Invasive Artificial Ventilation*,
DOI: 10.1007/978-88-470-5526-1_8, © Springer-Verlag Italia 2014

Fig. 8.1 The "journey" of
the central respiratory
impulse

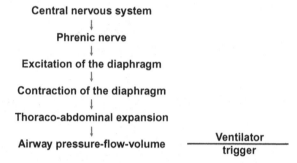

Central nervous system
↓
Phrenic nerve
↓
Excitation of the diaphragm
↓
Contraction of the diaphragm
↓
Thoraco-abdominal expansion
↓
Airway pressure-flow-volume

$$\frac{\text{Ventilator}}{\text{trigger}}$$

Preliminary physiological studies have demonstrated how good this method is with respect to, for example, pressure support ventilation. However, it remains unclear whether and, if so, how NAVA can improve clinical outcomes and how much the improvement of the patient/ventilator interaction also during NIV, may change the clinical history. We would, however, like to point out that NAVA requires the introduction of an esophageal catheter, a procedure which is actually invasive, and so it is somewhat a contradiction to the principle of a non invasive method of ventilation.

8.2   Airway Pressure-Release Ventilation or Biphasic Positive Airway Pressure

Be careful! This method, which is currently popular in some German-speaking countries, was originally called airway pressure-release ventilation (APRV) and more recently is also called biphasic positive airway pressure (BiPAP). It must not be confused with the BiPAP ventilator, which enables bilevel ventilation, that is Pressure Support + CPAP/external PEEP. APRV, or BiPAP®, has so far only be used in intubated patients with hypoxic respiratory failure as an alternative to volume ventilation. It consists of two levels of CPAP which are applied for a given period of time between which the patient can breathe spontaneously exactly as if with a single CPAP. However, unlike this latter, during APRV the operator may regulate the I:E ratio and the respiratory rate; thus, if the patient is not breathing spontaneously, it is indistinguishable from pressure-controlled ventilation. The tidal volume depends on the patient's compliance and resistances and on the difference in pressure between the two levels of CPAP.

8.3   High Frequency Ventilation

This term is used for some modes of ventilation characterized by tidal volumes lower than the anatomical dead space and with frequencies between 60 and 3,000 cycles per minute. Some of these, such as high frequency jet ventilation, are applied with a semi-invasive system.

- *High frequency positive pressure ventilation* (HFPPV). This mode is conceptually identical to intermittent positive pressure ventilation, which uses low tidal volumes and high frequencies (between 60 and 100 cycles/min);
- *High frequency jet ventilation* (HFJV). During this form of ventilation a small catheter is placed in the central airways, guaranteeing a supply of gas at a frequency of 60–240 cycles/min. The inspiratory time is set at about 20–50 % of the total respiratory time, while it is not possible to preset the patient's tidal volume because the volume delivered by the ventilator is the sum of that supplied by the machine and that actively produced by the patient;
- *High frequency oscillation.* This mode of ventilation consists of a very small tidal volume (1–3 mL/Kg) supplied by a high frequency piston (500–3,000 cycles/min). The gas is introduced using a flow system, while a small tube deals with the removal of CO_2;
- *Intrapulmonary percussive ventilation* (IPV). This is the only one of these methods applied non invasively with the main aim of removing bronchial secretions and improving the conditions so that the patient can undergo a cycle of NIV according to traditional dictates. As for HFPPV, IPV guarantees small volumes at high frequencies. For example, the "phasitron" system, working like a piston Venturi system, supported by compressed gas at a pressure from 0.8 to 3.5 bar, can generate from 80 to 650 cycles/min. IPV is indicated above all in patients with collections of secretions and difficulty in removing these secretions. We all know that the inability to eliminate bronchial secretions is one of the major limitations to the use of NIV but, as demonstrated in some studies, IPV could resolve this problem, restoring the conditions necessary for a trial of NIV. Nevertheless, it is important that the patient has a cough reflex, even if minimal, since it will be no help moving the secretions toward the oropharynx if the patient cannot then eliminate them. These devices, including an *in-exsufflator,* are also useful for chronic application in those neuromuscular pathologies in which weakness of the respiratory muscles makes it very difficult to eliminate secretions.

With the exception of IPV, the clinical use of these modes is limited because they seem to offer few advantages over the traditional techniques with regards to cardiovascular performance, intrapulmonary fluid accumulation, and gas exchange. The only fields of application are, therefore, limited to ventilation during bronchoscopy, laryngeal surgery, and the treatment of broncho-pleural fistulae that are proving resistant to closure. One further very interesting use that has given excellent clinical results is in the prevention of the development of chronic lung disease in premature babies and in those with neonatal bronchopulmonary dysplasia.

8.4   Volume-Assured Pressure Support Ventilation and Volume-Guaranteed Ventilation

This is a mode that has been almost completely abandoned in the intensive care unit, but has recently had a certain success during NIV, particularly in patients ventilated at home. Theoretically, the "real" volume assured pressure support ventilation (VAPS) combines the benefits of both pressure and volume ventilation. The operator decides the level of pressure support, a minimal tidal volume to reach and a peak inspiratory flow. During the first inspiratory phase, the algorithm of the ventilator extrapolates from the flow signal an estimated ideal volume that the patient will reach. If this is less than the minimum tidal volume, the ventilator supplies, within the same breath, the difference (Δ) in the volume needed to reach the target.

The major limit that we see in this algorithm concerns the calculation of the target volume based on the inspiratory flow which, as we know can increase in the presence of losses and therefore affect the calculation of the minimum guaranteed tidal volume, overestimating its value. In contrast, with ventilators for NIV or those for home use, the mechanism for integrating the volume is based on a progressive increase of pressure support. This particular type of ventilation can also be called volume-guaranteed ventilation. In other words, if the minimum volume is not reached for a few consecutive breaths, the ventilator will supply progressively increasing inspiratory pressures (up to a certain established upper limit), until the volume is raised above this threshold value. However, if the patient is able to generate a volume greater than the maximum established one, the ventilator will work in a different way, that is, gradually decreasing the inspiratory support. The advantage of these methods is that of theoretically ensuring effective ventilation in terms of tidal volume; the major disadvantage is that as the patient's clinical conditions change, he could need a greater minute volume. In this case, at least with some machines, the pressure support is reduced in response to an increased tidal volume, thus contrasting the patient's efforts to increase his ventilation. The ability of these modes of ventilation to compensate for non-intentional leaks depends, however, strictly on whether a "vented" (i.e., a non-rebreathing valve) or "non-vented" (true expiratory valve) circuit configuration is used. This difference must be taken into account as a possible risk when these modes are used with a "non-vented" circuit.

Suggested Reading

Amato MB, Barbas SC, Bonassa J et al (1992) Volume-assured pressure support ventilation (VAPSV). A new approach for reducing muscle workload during acute respiratory failure. Chest 102(4):1225–1234

Beamer WC, Prough DS, Royster RL et al (1984) High-frequency jet ventilation produces auto-PEEP. Crit Care Med 12(9):734–737

Cammarota G et al (2011) Noninvasive ventilation through a helmet in post extubation hypoxemic patients: physiologic comparison between neurally adjusted ventilatory assist and pressure support ventilation. Intensive Care Med 37:1943–1950

Carlon GC, Miodownik S, Ray C Jr, Kahn RC (1981) Technical aspects and clinical implications of high frequency jet ventilation with a solenoid valve. Crit Care Med 9(1):47–50

Carlucci A et al (2013) The configuration of bi-level ventilator circuits may affect compensation for non-intentional leaks during volume-targeted ventilation. Intensive Care Med 39(1):59–65

Courtney SE, Durand DJ, Asselin JM et al (2002) High-Frequency oscillatory ventilation versus conventional mechanical ventilation for very-low-birth-weight infants. New Engl J Med 347(9):643–652

Froese AB, Bryan AC (1987) High frequency ventilation. Am Rev Respir Dis 135(6):1363–1374

Jaber S, Delay JM, Matecki S (2005) Volume-guaranteed pressure support ventilation facing acute changes in ventilatory demand. Intensive Care Med 31(9):1181–1188

Lucangelo U, Antonaglia V, Zin WA (2004) Effects of mechanical load on flow, volume and pressure delivered by high-frequency percussive ventilation. Respir Physiol Neurobiol 142(1):81–91

Navalesi P, Costa R (2003) New modes of mechanical ventilation: proportional assist ventilation, neurally adjusted ventilatory assist and fractal ventilation. Curr Opin Crit Care 9(1):51–58

Putensen C, Wrigge H (2004) Clinical review: biphasic positive airway pressure and airway pressure release ventilation. Crit Care 8(6):492–497

Why is NIV Good?

9

Why should a relatively more complicated and perhaps more costly technique be better than intubation? We think that the answer is simple: NIV avoids most of the side effects of oro- or naso-tracheal intubation. By minimizing these complications we reduce on the one hand the time spent in hospital and on the other hand (but how difficult it is to explain this concept to our administrators) both hospital costs and "social" ones. All of this does, of course, have a human price to pay, which is changing normal practice, at least in some wards, learning something new and finally, perhaps, devoting more care to the patient in terms of time that doctors and paramedical staff spend at the patient's bedside.

NIV is, however, good. First of all, we reduce the need for neuromuscular blockade and sedation; although these can be considered convenient practices (the patient doesn't complain…), they do considerably prolong the period of ventilation and, therefore, the time spent in hospital.

Despite the efforts made to improve preventive measures, pneumonia associated with intubation, and not with the ventilation (!), complicates the prognosis in about 30 % of patients ventilated invasively. However, unlike infectious complications in other districts (e.g., urinary tract or skin), which are associated with a mortality rate ranging between 1 and 4 %, the mortality rate among patients who develop pneumonia is as high as 40–60 %. As we have just said, all this occurs despite recent improvements in diagnostics and potential treatments, in particular broad-spectrum antibiotics. This high mortality rate is due in part to a change in the population of patients admitted to intensive care units over the last 20 years, with an increase in elderly and more severely ill patients, and in part because of the proliferation of invasive diagnostic procedures, massive surgical interventions, and the introduction of immunosuppressive therapy. Those patients who develop pneumonia but manage to survive stay significantly longer in hospital, with their admission prolonged about threefold, which has a major impact on costs. The main causes of the high incidence of pneumonia include:

S. Nava and F. Fanfulla, *Non Invasive Artificial Ventilation*,
DOI: 10.1007/978-88-470-5526-1_9, © Springer-Verlag Italia 2014

- use of antibiotics (with the development of bacterial resistance);
- presence of an endotracheal tube, which increases the possibility aspirating pathogens and of local inflammatory lesions;
- presence of a nasogastric tube;
- enteral nutrition;
- supine position;
- massive surgery.

Controlled studies have clearly established that the incidence of nosocomial pneumonia is lower among patients ventilated non invasively than among those managed with invasive ventilation.

The essential condition for delivering invasive ventilation therapy is intubation, through either the mouth or nose. The frequency of complications related to this procedure is perhaps higher than commonly thought; indeed retrospective studies have quantified the incidence as being around >50 %. These complications can be divided essentially into those due to the act of intubation, those due to the presence of the tube *in situ* and those due to extubation.

The first group includes bleeding in the oral cavity or nose, dental trauma, excoriations, submucosal bleeding of the pharynx, edema, vocal cord lesions, arytenoid dislocation, tracheal perforation, and intubation of the right bronchus.

The complications related to the presence of the tube are skin reactions to the adhesive tape that keeps it in place, sinusitis, rhinorrhea, ear infections, and pressure sores in the pharynx and larynx which may become true ulcers.

The trachea is logically the most common site of lesions such as edema, ulcers, granulomas, submucosal hemorrhages, necrosis, cartilage destruction, dilatation, tracheomalacia, tracheo-esophageal fistulas, squamous metaplasia, reduced mucociliary clearance, and colonization of the airways.

The complications related to extubation are usually consequences of preexisting lesions, in particular stridor, paralysis and paresis of the vocal cords, cricoid abscesses, and the formation of adhesions.

As far as concerns lung damage induced by the ventilator, be this barotrauma, volutrauma, or biotrauma, it is not known whether NIV really reduces the occurrence of these complications even if, in daily clinical practice, we very rarely see cases of pneumothorax in patients undergoing NIV, but this could also depend on the severity of illness differing between patients ventilated invasively or non invasively.

Finally, problems related to the mechanism of swallowing should not be overlooked, since these often occur following placement of an endotracheal and/or tracheostomy tube.

Suggested Reading

Chastre J (1994) Pneumonia in the ventilator-dependent patient. In: Tobin M (ed) Principles and practice of mechanical ventilation. McGraw-Hill, New York

Craven DE, Kunches LM, Kilinsky V et al (1986) Risk factors for pneumonia and fatality in patients receiving continuous mechanical ventilation. Am Rev Respir Dis 133(5):792–796

Elpern EH, Scott MG, Petro L, Ries MH (1994) Pulmonary aspiration in mechanically ventilated patients with tracheostomies. Chest 105(2):563–566

Epstein SK (2006) Complications associated with mechanical ventilation. In: Tobin MJ (ed) Principles and practice of mechanical ventilation, 2nd edn. McGraw-Hill, New York

Fagon JY, Chastre J, Domart Y et al (1989) Nosocomial pneumonia in patients receiving continuous mechanical ventilation, prospective analysis of 52 episodes with use of a protected specimen brush and quantitative culture techniques. Am Rev Respir Dis 139(4):877–884

Fagon JY, Chastre J, Hance AJ et al (1993) Nosocomial pneumonia in ventilated patients: a cohort study evaluating attributable mortality and hospital stay. Am J Med 94(3):281–288

Girou E, Schortgen F, Delcalux C et al (2000) Association of noninvasive ventilation with nosocomial infections and survival in critically ill patients. JAMA 284(18):2361–2367

Le Bourdelles G, Viires N, Boczkowski J et al (1994) Effects of mechanical ventilation on diaphragmatic contractile properties in rats. Am J Respir Crit Care Med 149(6):1539–1544

Martin LF, Booth FV, Reines HD et al (1992) Stress ulcers and organ failure in intubated patients in surgical intensive care units. Ann Surg 215(4):332–337

Ranieri VM, Giunta F, Suter PM, Slutsky AS (2000) Mechanical ventilation as a mediator of multisystem organ failure in acute respiratory distress syndrome. JAMA 284(1):43–44

Shapiro M, Wilson RK, Casar G et al (1986) Work of breathing through different sized endotracheal tubes. Crit Care Med 14(12):1028–3101

Stauffer JL et al (1981) Complications and consequences of endotracheal intubation and tracheostomy. Am J Med 70:65–76

Myths, Prejudices and Real Problems 10

This chapter focuses, in no particular order, on some common place ideas that positively or negatively often limit the use of NIV or, on the other hand, overestimate its therapeutic properties.

10.1 The Side Effects are Negligible

We must clarify immediately that although the side effects of NIV are much less dramatic than those of intubation, they absolutely must not be underestimated because they sometimes determine whether or not the method is tolerated. They can, therefore, automatically become a cause of failed NIV and intubation, which may sometimes be delayed, is consequently more hazardous.

Intolerance to and poor compliance with the interface are real problems during NIV, but can be mitigated by a careful choice of the mask and mode of ventilation, assuming that the patient is cooperative.

Table 10.1 shows that the most serious and most common side effect is nasal lesions, which are superficially dismissed in numerous studies as "nasal reddening." While it is true that this is the only sign present in most patients, it is well known that some individuals develop much more serious lesions that can lead in some cases to total necrosis of the nasal bridge and, consequently, immediate suspension of the ventilation therapy.

There are scales, such as the one shown in Table 10.2, which can be used to monitor pressure sores, similar to those use for major bedsores (e.g., sacral pressure sores), which we should accustom ourselves to using. These lesions are caused by the excessive pressure exerted by the mask in an attempt to prevent air losses: the lack of an adequate circulation below the mask leads first to reddening and then, in some cases, to necrosis. Prevention consists of applying protections, such as those used around abdominal stoma, on the part of the nose in contact with the mask or of trying to minimize the pressure by applying reinforcements to the masks, which should keep the apex of the device lifted away from the skin.

S. Nava and F. Fanfulla, *Non Invasive Artificial Ventilation*,
DOI: 10.1007/978-88-470-5526-1_10, © Springer-Verlag Italia 2014

Table 10.1 Side effects of
NIV described in the
literature

• Due to the interface	Frequency (%)
- Discomfort	30–50
- Facial erythema	20–30
- Claustrophobia	5–10
- Nasal ulcers	5–10
- Skin rash	5–10
• Due to the flow of air	
- Nasal congestion	20–50
- Sinusitis	10–30
- Dry mouth	10–20
- Ocular irritation	10–20
- Gastric distension	5–10
• Air leaks	80–100
• Severe complications	
- Aspiration pneumonia	<5
- Hypotension	<5
- Pneumothorax	<5

It is very often believed that fixing the interface very tightly to the patient's face will reduce air losses to a minimum. This is not exactly true, given that in one *in vitro* study it was demonstrated that it is the difference between the pressure applied by the cushion surrounding the structure of the mask and the pressure of insufflation of the ventilator, which determines the amount of air loss. Figure 10.1 shows that, according to this study, there is no point in increasing the difference between these two pressures to over 2 cmH_2O, since above this value the loss remains constant and limited, even though the operator obstinately continues to

Table 10.2 Classification of nasal pressure sores. Adapted from the European pressure ulcer advisory panel, guidelines 1998

GRADE 0: absent

GRADE 1: intact skin with or without erythema. Induration of the skin with slight edema are indicators in dark-skinned individuals

GRADE 2: partial thickness skin loss involving epidermis, dermis, or both. The ulcer is superficial and presents clinically as an abrasion or blister

GRADE 3: substantial loss of tissue with damage to or necrosis of subcutaneous tissue that does not involve the muscle fascia

GRADE 4: extensive tissue destruction with necrosis or direct damage to muscle, cartilage, or supporting structures increase the pressure against the surface of the nose. We should also remember that NIV is by definition a semi-open system so, when using a good ventilator, small losses are tolerated.

After a few hours of ventilation, patients may also complain of rhinorrhea or, contrariwise, excessive dryness of the nose and throat, which requires the use of a humidification system (see later). Pooled secretions may block the nasal passages, which can interfere with the ventilation, but this problem is easily resolved by nasal lavages with water or by using, with caution, ephedrine drops.

Another side effect of NIV is gastric distension which can be particularly annoying when it prevents correct expansion of the abdomen during inspiration or when the patients is not breathing in harmony with the ventilator. However, this side effect is uncommon, even though North American authors highlight this as one of the most frequent problems occurring during NIV. In some cases, it can be circumvented by reducing the pressure of insufflation or the time of pressurization.

There is a risk of hyperventilation, particularly during the night, in neuro-muscular patients, in whom the impedance of the system is particularly low and in whom the $PaCO_2$ can drop abruptly, causing acute closure of the glottis to prevent hypocapnia. The mechanism can lead to the onset of episodes of central apnea.

Precisely because patients receiving NIV are rarely sedated, their sleep may be fairly disturbed. One practical tip is to reduce the ventilator's alarms to a minimum and, if the patient is admitted to a subintensive therapy unit, to move him to a traditional ward as soon as his clinical conditions allow.

The side effect of reddened eyes is fairly common, particularly if the insufflation pressures are high; we must remember to take particular care in protecting the eyes when administering nebulized anticholinergics through the NIV circuit, given that phenomena of anisocoria have been observed. As said earlier, all these problems are minor side effects, but can have a substantial influence on the

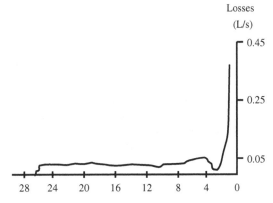

Fig. 10.1 The effect of mask fixation pressure on air leaks. Modified from Schettino et al. (2001)

Losses (L/s)

Occlusion pressure (mask fixation pressure – airway pressure) (cmH$_2$O)

tolerance to NIV and thereby lead to its failure. This is why the operator must devote great care to minimizing or preventing these problems.

10.2   NIV Does Not Work in Severely Ill Patients

We will deal with the clinical effects of NIV in the specific chapters. Here we will concentrate on the common criticism, raised particularly by our intensive care colleagues, that NIV should be reserved only for less severely ill patients and, therefore, as prevention of intubation rather than as a real alternative. However, 10–15 years ago, it was said that NIV would never enter intensive care, whereas it is now the method used by 50 % of ventilated patients in some countries, such as France.

That said, we do agree with the fact that using NIV in some particularly ill patients, especially if they have acute hypoxic respiratory failure, would definitely be imprudent. For example, it has been demonstrated that sepsis, hemodynamic instability and shock, the presence of ARDS and the lack of improvement in the PaO_2/FiO_2 after <1 h of NIV are inversely correlated with the success of NIV. We should all remember the fundamental concept of medicine, which is "first do no harm," meaning that a brief, judicious trial of NIV can be attempted, but always bearing in mind that the worst problem that we could cause is culpably delaying intubation. One of the key factors for NIV in hypoxic respiratory failure is therefore its early use, when the clinical conditions have still not deteriorated too much. In other words, "the earlier you start, the better are your chances of success".

We must, however, also appreciate that there are conditions, such as exacerbations of COPD and acute pulmonary edema, for which the use of NIV or CPAP is the "first-line" treatment independently of the severity of the patient's clinical condition. It is clear, and we have demonstrated it in the past, that the success of NIV depends on the experience of the team. Indeed, over time, and with a fairly prolonged training period, patients can be treated successfully who would previously have been destined to failure if managed by the same team in the same hospital (Fig. 10.2). In any case, some studies have shown that even in COPD patients with very severe acidosis (pH < 7.22) intubation is not superior to NIV in improving clinical outcome and, indeed, that this latter is associated with fewer side effects and a lesser need for tracheotomy.

10.3   The Work Load Necessary for NIV is Too Onerous

One of the greatest limitations to the generalized use of NIV is the prejudice that this technique is associated with excessive expenditure of human resources. While it is certainly true that one does not become experienced and expert in the field from 1 day to another, it is equally true that after acquiring a bit of theory and

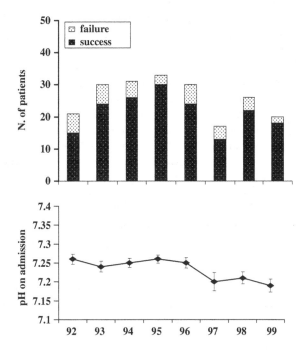

Fig. 10.2 Reduction in the rate of NIV failure over the years, despite increasing severity of respiratory failure. Modified from Carlucci et al. (2003)

practice, using appropriate equipment and being aware of one's own limits, particularly at the beginning, a good NIV service can be established. This is the right place to point out that NIV is never the skill of a single person, but the work of a team whose operative efficacy must always be periodically checked by audits. Let's remember this fact and involve all the members of the team: nurses, physiotherapists, and doctors.

The myth that NIV is onerous in human terms has a very precise origin. In 1991, Chevrolet et al. published one of the most frequently cited papers on NIV in the literature, since it reported the results of the first study designed to determine the human costs of this sort of ventilation therapy. The title itself rings as a warning to anyone who wants to try this technique: "Nasal positive pressure ventilation in patients with acute respiratory failure. Difficult and time-consuming procedure for nurses". The results of this study were surprising given that the authors quantified that the time necessary for the care of COPD patients during NIV was 91 % of the total time of ventilation, whereas this time dropped to 41 % in patients with restrictive airway diseases. The limitations of the study, which were substantial, are well-known: the observational and, therefore, not controlled nature of the study, the small number of patients and, above all, the paucity of the group's training and experience. Indeed, 10 years later, the same authors demonstrated that, with the acquisition of greater confidence and more experience, the previously found unacceptable times and difficulties had been drastically reduced. This is in line with many other studies concordantly stating that while NIV is indeed more time-consuming than traditional medicine in the first hours of treatment, this effect then disappears, and the patients' clinical outcome is better. The opening of subintensive respiratory care units has certainly helped to overturn the traditional view of the management of ventilated patients, since the medical and paramedical staff in these units are experts in the treatment of both intubated and non invasively ventilated patients.

Since NIV remains not only a method of prevention, but also a real alternative to intubation, it is important to remember that when direct comparisons of human time expenditure for NIV and invasive ventilation are made, the times have been found not to differ greatly. Comparing these two groups of patients, the time of care by the whole hospital staff in the first 24 h was not significantly different between the two groups and remained below 50 % of the total time of ventilation. A detailed analysis of the times, divided according to the type of healthcare professional, showed that the time employed by nurses and rehabilitation therapists decreased significantly after the first 6 h of ventilation, reaching a plateau, whereas the amount of time dedicated to the patient by medical staff remained constant for the first 48 h.

We can, therefore, dismantle the prejudice concerning the difficulties of administering NIV, stating that, at least in specialist environments, this form of ventilation does not seem to affect the time expenditure and workloads of the hospital staff significantly.

Obviously, the management of non invasively ventilated patients is more complicated in hospital wards in which the staff are not familiar with the method of NIV and for this reason it could indeed still be more time-consuming in settings such as intensive care.

10.4 The Helmet is the Interface of Choice

This is the typical statement of some colleagues who have a rather short memory. NIV originated decades ago as a technique that used exclusively nasal or oro-nasal interfaces. The most impressive results from both clinical and scientific points of view were obtained with these masks, such that, to our knowledge, there are no randomized controlled studies on the use of the helmet.

That said, we must all be open to new technology. The helmet has certainly simplified the application of CPAP outside protected environments. Its ease of use avoiding electric sockets, setting the parameters, the irritation of alarms, the good tolerance that patients report when ventilated with this interface and, finally, the low cost due to the possibility of administering a form of NIV without buying a ventilator have made this the interface of choice for the treatment acute pulmonary edema outside hospitals or in unspecialized wards. None of this detracts from the fact that CPAP administered by a helmet can also be used successfully in intensive care.

The huge popularity of this interface during the application of "true" NIV is concentrated particularly in Italy, where it has become the first choice in intensive care. As already specified in the section on interfaces, the helmet is associated with problems of patient-ventilator synchrony (even when particular settings are adopted), difficulty with humidification, and noise but, above all, must be used with extreme care in hypercapnic patients because of the large dead space. Having said this, a helmet can be a valid alternative to face masks in the case that these latter are poorly tolerated, or in the context of rotating different types of interfaces during the daytime hours of ventilation in order to avoid some specific side effects of each of the interfaces.

In our opinion, the helmet is certainly not the interface of first choice and its use in Europe (<10 % of patients ventilated non invasively) shows this.

10.5   It is Better Not to Use an Interface with a Large Dead Space

A large dead space is associated with the concept of a large volume within the interface itself. For this reason, the bulkier masks, such as the total face and the full mask, are often viewed with a certain skepticism. Years ago, we demonstrated that the *in vitro* dead space, that is, the volume measured by filling a mask with water, is not necessarily the same as the *in vitro* dead space, when the mask is applied to a patient's face. The notable difference in dead space found *in vitro* between a nasal mask and a facial mask is not, therefore, present when the measurements are made *in vitro*. Not long ago, Fraticelli et al. (2009) demonstrated that when it came to improving gas exchange, and removal of CO_2 in particular, there was no difference between four interfaces that had considerably different dead spaces, for example, a mouthpiece (dead space of 0 ml) and a total face mask (dead space of 977 ml). However, for the same efficacy, ventilation via a mouthpiece was associated with an increased incidence of asynchrony between the patient and ventilator. One rather particular case is the helmet, which requires a high flow of oxygen to avoid the well-recognized problem of rebreathing. In conclusion, do not be afraid of a dead space effect when using a facial ventilation interface with a large internal volume.

10.6   A Patient Being Non Invasively Ventilated Must Not Be Sedated

The possibility and appropriateness of sedating a patient during NIV is one of the most widely debated problems. Theoretically, NIV should only be applied to subjects who have some minimum residual autonomous respiration and are, therefore, able to trigger the ventilator. Furthermore, one of the presumed advantages of NIV is that of not requiring neuromuscular blockade or profound sedation. However, in clinical practice, we can find ourselves faced with very anxious and irritable patients who rebel against the interface and often try to remove it. What should we do in these situations? Should we risk further limiting the capacity to breathe spontaneously and end up having to intubate the patient urgently or debunk a little bit the myth that sedatives always and in any case interfere with the respiratory drive? The indications, the preferred drug, and the doses of sedatives to administer are all currently under study.

What is known, however, is that sedation is actually being used in the real world even during NIV. A survey of North Americans and Europeans found that the practice of sedation varied enormously in relation to geography, type of structure in which the NIV was applied and the type of specialist prescribing it. Surprisingly, one of the most widely used methods in North America is that of tying the patients' hands to the bed, a somewhat cruel and ethically debatable practice in our opinion, and fortunately much less used in Europe, except in the most difficult cases.

The most widely used drugs in North America are benzodiazepines alone, followed by opioids (morphine and fentanyl), while exactly the opposite is the case in Europe. Our experience with benzodiazepines has not always been positive since, although there are specific antidotes, side effects (e.g., hemodynamic decompensation) are not uncommon in the elderly and are not always easily neutralized by the antagonists. Haloperidol is also used with a certain frequency, although in intensive care it tends to be reserved particularly for delirious patients taking into account its possible side effects, which may be severe, such a *torsades de pointes*. Dexemetomidine, on the other hand, is rarely used, perhaps because of its high costs, despite being probably the only compound that has been found not to have side effects on the central nervous system even when given for more than 24 h. The use of sedation is almost never based on specific protocols but rather on the physician's experience; the preferred route of administration is extemporaneous boluses. One of the most interesting findings of the survey was that the frequency of use of sedatives and analgesics was proportional to the use of NIV in a given setting, as if more expert staff had fewer qualms about giving drugs. All things considered, the most widely used doses for NIV are within the safe range, since there are no published studies demonstrating a clear effect of benzodiazepines and opioids on respiratory drive at these doses. Our advice is to record the patient's level of sedation using the Ramsey scale (Table 10.3).

Table 10.3 Ramsay sedation score. Modified from Hansen-Flaschen et al. (1994)

1	Patient anxious and agitated
2	Patient cooperative, oriented and calm
3	Patient responsive to commands only
4	Patient responds briskly to glabellar compression
5	Patient responds sluggishly to glabellar compression
6	Patient unresponsive to glabellar compression

Interesting pilot studies can help us to give some clinical advice. In two studies in patients who had failed an initial trial of NIV because of intolerance, it was demonstrated that the use of a new opioid based on anilidopiperidine (rimifentanil) was able to avoid the need for intubation in nine of them (69 %). The starting dose used was 0.025 µg/kg/min, given intravenously, and then the dose was increased up to a maximum of 0.15 µg/kg, until reaching a sedation score between two and three on the Ramsey scale. In three patients in whom the maximum dose was reached, propofol had to be added.

In conclusion, our advice is that "judicious" sedation should not be denied before declaring NIV a total failure in an agitated patient and, therefore, intubating the patient immediately.

10.7   It is (Almost) Impossible to Use NIV in a Comatose Patient

As a joke to disprove this statement, it could be said that it is easier to ventilate comatose patients, particularly if their sensorial dulling is based on hypercapnia, than it is to ventilate to over-agitated patients. If anything, the problems could start later, when the patient wakes up!

An altered sensorium has always been considered an absolute or relative contraindication to NIV in guidelines and state-of-the-art conferences. What do we mean by sensorial dulling? The classical scales used in neurological settings, such as the Glasgow Coma Scale, are of little help in patients with respiratory disorders, whereas the Kelly scale for monitoring the state of consciousness is certainly more appropriate for our patients. This simple instrument, presented in Table 5.2, enables the level of consciousness to be classified with sufficient precision. In most of the studies carried out, only patients with a score of 1 or 2 were ventilated with NIV. A series of case-controlled studies compared the outcomes of patients with COPD and an intact sensorium with those of a group of stuporous patients who could only carry out simple commands after "vigorous" attempts at arousal (grade > 2). The probability of failure of NIV was undoubtedly higher in this latter group of patients, but certainly better than could have been expected and over 50 %. With due caution it is, therefore, advisable not to exclude patients with sensorial dulling *a priori* from a trial with NIV, taking into account that this should only be performed in a protected environment in which intubation can be performed promptly and, in particular, focusing on those patients whose encephalopathy is due to severe hypercapnia.

10.8   Reimbursement for NIV Through the DRG System

More than a myth or a prejudice, reimbursement for NIV through the DRG System is a real problem. But how much does NIV cost? The direct costs are defined as the expenses necessary to evaluate and treat the individual patient and, therefore, include functional studies and tests (for example, X-rays, blood-gas analyses), the costs of drugs and disposable equipment (for example, masks and tubes), and salaries of the medical and paramedical staff. The cost of the staff per patient is usually derived by multiplying the number of days in hospital by the daily wage for each component of the staff involved in the care of the patient. For example, if the doctor–patient ratio in an intensive respiratory unit is 1:3, the cost for a patient admitted for 10 days is calculated by multiplying the daily wage (gross) of a doctor by 10 and dividing by three. The costs of the disposable equipment used by the staff to treat the patients (masks, gloves, etc.) must then be added to the previously calculated direct costs.

Indirect hospital costs are those costs necessary to cover the institute's services, such as heating, laundry, transport, administrative staff, amortization of equipment (ventilators, monitoring systems), and many others.

A study by Kramer et al. demonstrated that in the 1990s the daily cost of NIV was USA dollars (USD) 1,850, equivalent to about €1,500, for an average period of admission of 20 days, while the daily cost of traditional medical therapy was USD 1,800, equivalent to about €1,450, for an average admission of 18 days (Kramer et al. 1995).

Criner and colleagues designed an *ad hoc* study to analyze costs, although the study did not include a control group. The daily cost of each of the patients treated with NIV was USD 1,570 (about €1,200) for a mean time of 20 days spent in hospital, thus essentially replicating the results obtained by Kramer (Criner et al. 1995).

In the study that we carried out to quantify medical and paramedical activity during NIV and invasive ventilation treatment, we analyzed overall costs using the same scheme as that used in the previously cited North American studies. The costs of the two ventilatory techniques were comparable, although considerably lower than those in the previously cited studies. The daily costs in the first 48 h of NIV were quantified as USD 806, equivalent to about €600, while those for invasive ventilation were USD 865, equivalent to €650 (Nava et al. 1997). Some years later, we calculated that the average daily cost could be reduced if the less severely ill patients (i.e., with a pH > 7.28) were treated in a ward. For example, compared with a daily cost of €558 of non invasively ventilating a patient with an exacerbation of COPD in a subintensive therapy unit, the same method used in a ward cost €470. These costs were calculated in a single structure, in which the medical ward considered was "physically" connected to the subintensive therapy unit (Carlucci et al. 2003).

It is clear that the impact of the diagnostic procedures, the drugs and equipment are similar in absolute terms, in either euros or dollars; what differed significantly was the salary of the staff, whether medical or paramedical.

The DRG reimbursement system is very punitive. Criner et al. calculated the loss due to this system of payment for 27 patients treated acutely in an intensive care unit. The mean time spent in hospital was about 20 days and the financial loss per patient was USD 9,700, with 82 % of the cases being under-reimbursed (Criner et al. 1995). In Italy too, the introduction of the DRG reimburesement system has clearly favored some practices (e.g., tracheotomy), but penalized others. At this point, if we have given scientific and clinical dignity to NIV as an alternative to invasive ventilation, we must now try to make it considered equivalent also from an economic point of view. It is ventilation in any case, simply with a different interface.

As far as concerns the cost-effectiveness ratio of NIV, there is no longer any doubt that this treatment drastically reduces expenses, at least for the treatment of patients with exacerbations of COPD. For example, Plant et al. demonstrated that about £54,000 could be saved annually by treating 56 patients in this way in a year in typical hospital in the United Kingdom (Plant et al. 2003).

Furthermore, the fact that infectious complications are less common with NIV than with invasive ventilation is another indirect cause of saving. A study published in *Public Health Report* (Klevens et al. 2007) showed that the total cost of a case of ventilator-associated pneumonia is more than USD 100,000 per patient. In the light of this, it was thought in the USA to consider ventilator-associated pneumonia as an avoidable complication and not, therefore, reimbursable by the agency responsible for hospital reimbursements. So here in another good occasion to use NIV, but also to sensitize the people pulling the wires of the national health system to consider a different form of reimbursement.

Suggested Reading

Agarwal R, Reddy C, Aggarwal AN, Gupta D (2006) Is there a role for noninvasive ventilation in acute respiratory distress syndrome? A meta-analysis. Respir Med 100(12):2235–2238

Ambrosino N, Vagheggini G (2008) Noninvasive positive pressure ventilation in the acute care setting: where are we? Eur Respir J 31(4):874–886

Antonelli M, Conti G, Pelosi P et al (2002) New treatment of acute hypoxemic respiratory failure: noninvasive pressure support ventilation delivered by helmet—a pilot controlled trial. Crit Care Med 30(3):602–608

Antonelli M, Conti G, Esquinas A (2007) A multiple-center survey on the use in clinical practice of noninvasive ventilation as a first-line intervention for acute respiratory distress syndrome. Crit Care Med 35(19):18–25

Carlucci A, Delmastro M, Rubini F (2003) Changes in the practice of non-invasive ventilation in treating COPD patients over 8 years. Intensive Care Med 29(3):419–425

Chevrolet JC, Jolliet P, Abajo B et al (1991) Nasal positive pressure ventilation in patients with acute respiratory failure. Difficult and time-consuming procedure for nurses. Chest 100(3):775–782

Constantin JM, Schneider E, Cayot-Constantin S et al (2007) Remifentanil-based sedation to treat noninvasive ventilation failure: a preliminary study. Intensive Care Med 33(1):82–87

Crimi C, Noto A, Princi P et al (2010) A European survey of non-invasive ventilation practices. Eur Respir J 36(2):362–369

Criner GJ, Kreimer DT, Tomaselli M et al (1995) Financial implications of noninvasive positive pressure ventilation (NPPV). Chest 108:475–481

Devlin JW, Nava S, Fong JJ et al (2007) Survey of sedation practices during noninvasive positive–pressure ventilation to treat acute respiratory failure. Crit Care Med 35(10):2298–2302

Esteban A, Ferguson ND, Meade MO et al (2008) Evolution of mechanical ventilation in response to clinical research. Am J Respir Crit Care Med 177(2):170–177

European Pressure Ulcer Advisory Panel (1998) Guidelines. http://www.epuap. org/gltreatment.html

Fodil R, Lellouche F, Mancebo J et al (2011) Comparison of patient–ventilator interfaces based on their computerized effective deadspace. Intensive Care Med 37:257–262

Fraticelli AT, Lellouche F, L'her E et al (2009) Physiological effects of different interfaces during noninvasive ventilation for acute respiratory failure. Crit Care Med 37(3):939–945

Hansen-Flaschen J, Cowen J, Polomano RC (1994) Beyond the Ramsay scale: need for a validated measure of sedating drug efficacy in the intensive care unit. Crit Care Med 22(5):732–733

Jolliet P, Abajo B, Pasquina P, Chevrolet JC (2001) Non-invasive pressure support ventilation in severe community-acquired pneumonia. Intensive Care Med 27(5):812–821

Klevens RM, Edwards JR, Richards CL Jr et al (2007) Estimating health care-associated infections and deaths in U.S. hospitals, 2002. Public Health Rep 122(2):160–166

Kramer N, Meyer TJ, Meharg J et al (1995) Randomized, prospective trial of noninvasive positive pressure ventilation in acute respiratory failure. Am J Respir Crit Care Med 151:1799–1806

Milan M, Zanella A, Isgro S et al (2011) Performance of different continuous positive airway pressure helmets equipped with safety valves during failure of fresh gas supply. Intensive Care Med 37:1031–1035

Nava S, Hill N (2009) Non-invasive ventilation in acute respiratory failure. Lancet 374(9685):250–259

Nava S, Evangelisti I, Rampulla C (1997) Human and financial costs of noninvasive mechanical ventilation in patients affected by COPD and acute respiratory failure. Chest 111(6):1631–1638

Navalesi P, Fanfulla F, Frigerio P et al (2000) Physiologic evaluation of noninvasive mechanical ventilation delivered with three types of masks in patients with chronic hypercapnic respiratory failure. Crit Care Med 28(6):1785–1790

Navalesi P, Costa R, Ceriana P et al (2007) Non-invasive ventilation in chronic obstructive pulmonary disease patients: helmet versus facial mask. Intensive Care Med 33(1):74–81

Plant PK, Owen JL, Parrott S, Elliott MW (2003) Cost effectiveness of ward based non-invasive ventilation for acute exacerbations of chronic obstructive pulmonary disease: economic analysis of randomised controlled trial. BMJ 326:956–961

Rocco M, Conti G, Alessandri E et al (2010) Rescue treatment for noninvasive ventilation failure due to interface intolerance with remifentanil analgosedation: a pilot study. Intensive Care Med 36:2060–2065

Schettino GP, Tucci MR, Sousa R et al (2001) Mask mechanics and leak dynamics during noninvasive pressure support ventilation: a bench study. Intensive Care Med 27(12):1887–1891

Taccone P, Hess D, Caironi P, Bigatello LM (2004) Continuous positive airway pressure delivered with a "helmet": effects on carbon dioxide rebreathing. Crit Care Med 32(10):2090–2096

Zhan Q, Sun B, Liang L et al (2012) Early use of noninvasive positive pressure ventilation for acute lung injury: A multicenter randomized controlled trial. Crit Care Med 40:455–460

NIV in the Treatment of Acute Respiratory Failure: The Magnificent Five

11

In the full flood of evidence-based medicine, whose contents we often do not actually agree with, it is now relative easy to organize a grading of the evidence on the indications for NIV, which we have listed according to the scheme proposed by the Oxford Centre for Evidence-based Medicine (Fig. 11.1).

According to this classification, there are the "magnificent five" indications for the use of NIV: exacerbation of COPD, acute pulmonary edema, pneumonia in immunocompromised patients, weaning the COPD patient from invasive ventilation and, finally, prevention of post-extubation respiratory failure in patients at risk.

The other clinical applications, although important and worthy of further study, have not yet been conferred the level of scientific evidence for which NIV is to be considered the gold standard management for those applications. This does not mean that NIV for these applications cannot be validated scientifically and—why not—tested in our clinical practice, but greater caution is required. We will deal with each one of the five confirmed indications separately.

11.1 Exacerbation of COPD

After the first uncontrolled, nonrandomized studies back at the end of the 1980s, during which the promising advantages of NIV already began to be seen, in the period between 1993 and 1998 there were five important randomized, controlled trials comparing the efficacy of NIV combined with standard medical therapy compared to standard medical therapy alone in the treatment of exacerbations of COPD. Four of these studies demonstrated the superiority of NIV, which was successful in more than 90 % of cases, compared to medical therapy alone, which had a maximum success rate of 70 % in the study by Bott and much lower rates in the other studies (Bott et al. 1993).

S. Nava and F. Fanfulla, *Non Invasive Artificial Ventilation*,
DOI: 10.1007/978-88-470-5526-1_11, © Springer-Verlag Italia 2014

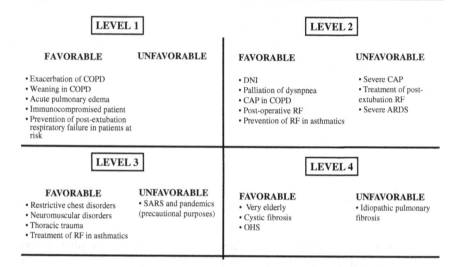

LEVEL 1		LEVEL 2	
FAVORABLE	**UNFAVORABLE**	**FAVORABLE**	**UNFAVORABLE**
• Exacerbation of COPD • Weaning in COPD • Acute pulmonary edema • Immunocompromised patient • Prevention of post-extubation respiratory failure in patients at risk		• DNI • Palliation of dysnpnea • CAP in COPD • Post-operative RF • Prevention of RF in asthmatics	• Severe CAP • Treatment of post-extubation RF • Severe ARDS
LEVEL 3		LEVEL 4	
FAVORABLE	**UNFAVORABLE**	**FAVORABLE**	**UNFAVORABLE**
• Restrictive chest disorders • Neuromuscular disorders • Thoracic trauma • Treatment of RF in asthmatics	• SARS and pandemics (precautional purposes)	• Very elderly • Cystic fibrosis • OHS	• Idiopathic pulmonary fibrosis

Fig. 11.1 Levels of scientific evidence: *LEVEL 1* systemic reviews based on randomized control trials with small confidence intervals; *LEVEL 2* reviews of single cohort studies, cohort studies or poorer quality randomized controlled trials; *LEVEL 3* reviews of case-controlled studies or individual case-controlled studies, *LEVEL 4* observational studies or case-controlled cohort studies of lesser quality

Only the study by Barbé et al. produced data that were discordant with these: in their study, the percentage success rates of NIV and medical therapy were 70 and 100 %, respectively (Barbé et al. 1996). This study, which was performed on patients with mild disease was mild, showed that NIV should be reserved to relatively compromised patients and should not, therefore, be used when medical treatment has a reasonable possibility of success and the NIV could be poorly tolerated by the patient.

This concept was clearly reaffirmed in a subsequent systematic review of the literature by Keenan, who showed that the efficacy of NIV is maximal in severe exacerbations of COPD (Keenan et al. 2003). Nevertheless, it is important to consider in what context the ventilator therapy is applied. For example, a multi-center randomized study by Plant et al. published in The Lancet and carried out in so-called "respiratory wards" showed that NIV was superior to medical therapy; however, a subsequent analysis showed that this effect too was explained by the high success rate among patients with a pH between 7.34 and 7.30 (Plant et al. 2000). The most severely ill patients did not have particularly satisfactory outcomes, and these were comparable to those obtained with traditional therapy.

As we said in the chapter, "When to start (or not) ventilation treatment" it is not only the timing of NIV, but also its place of use, that is fundamental in determining whether the therapy will be a failure or success. In other words, although the various reviews suggest that the success rate of NIV during an exacerbation of COPD is high also among patients with a pH < 7.30, we must bear in mind that many of the studies considered were carried out in protected environments (*i.e.* intensive or subintensive care units) and that these results should not be generalized to classical respiratory or general medicine wards without considering the staff, structure, monitoring, and ventilators available in such wards. In conclusion, compared to medical treatment alone, in patients with an exacerbation of COPD, NIV improves survival, reduces the need for intubation, lowers the rate of complications and shortens the time spent in intensive care and in hospital.

All the studies on the efficacy of NIV considered so far compared this method with standard medical therapy, in part because the purpose of NIV was usually prevention of endotracheal intubation and not as an alternative to it. The only two clinical studies in which the two methods of ventilation, invasive and non invasive, are compared were performed in Italy and Croatia.

In a study by Conti and colleagues in 2002 (Conti et al. 2002), a group of patients were admitted to the intensive care unit because of acute hypercapnic respiratory failure resulting from an exacerbation of COPD (mean pH, 7.21) after failure of standard medical treatment in the emergency department, so with an elective indication for ventilatory support. The patients were randomized to treatment with invasive or non invasive ventilation. The outcome of the two groups was comparable; they had the same improvement in blood gases, duration of ventilation, time spent in hospital, and number of complications. About 50 % of the NIV group avoided intubation. A follow-up carried out 1 year later revealed that the patients in the NIV group had required fewer hospital admissions and prescriptions of home oxygen therapy. This study confirmed that patients with more severe blood-gas disturbances should be treated in the intensive care unit, in order that they can be intubated immediately if the NIV fails. In the Croatian study, the duration of mechanical ventilation was overall 78 h shorter in the NIV group, and the time spent in the intensive care unit was also reduced. Ventilator-associated pneumonia occurred in 6 % and 37 % of the NIV group and intubated group, respectively.

In another case-controlled study, Squadrone and colleagues (Squadrone et al. 2004) recruited patients with hypercapnic respiratory failure due to an acute exacerbation of COPD or pneumonia with a mean pH of 7.18. The NIV failed in 60 % of the patients who were then intubated. The mortality, duration of mechanical ventilation, and length of hospital stay were similar in the two groups of patients, but the patients treated with NIV had fewer complications.

NIV is, therefore, undoubtedly the first-line treatment for exacerbations of COPD, provided that the patient does not have any of the classical contraindications to the method. This should now be standard practice in our wards; although it unfortunately sometimes still occurs, it is no longer acceptable to deny these patients ventilation treatment *a priori* with the excuse of age, number of past exacerbations or, worse still, the impossibility of finding a bed.

11.2   Acute Pulmonary Edema

The treatment of acute, cardiogenic pulmonary edema with NIV deserves a section apart. From a physiological point of view, the application of a positive pressure has beneficial effects on both respiration and hemodynamics.

In particular, continuous positive pressure such as CPAP increases residual functional capacity, thereby improving lung compliance and, consequently, oxygenation. The decreased respiratory work load resulting from the administration of CPAP, particularly the reduction in deflections of pleural pressure, leads to a decrease in transmural pressure of the left ventricle which, in turn, reduces the preload, thereby improving hemodynamics, which are severely compromised during acute pulmonary edema. Is there any sense adding inspiratory support (i.e., Pressure Support) to the CPAP? From a physiological point of view, the combination of the two pressures could have a rationale when the patient not only has hypoxia but also hypercapnia, which, it should be recalled, is the sign of ventilatory pump impairment. In these conditions, inspiratory support could further reduce the load against which the respiratory muscles contract, thus avoiding respiratory distress and the potential onset of fatigue.

From a clinical point of view, numerous meta-analyses have shown that CPAP combined with medical therapy is more effective than oxygen therapy associated with medical therapy in reducing the need for intubation and, above all, in improving survival. Medical therapy should not, however, be suspended because the reason for any form of CPAP or other ventilatory support is to "gain time" until the nitrates and any diuretics prescribed can act.

CPAP delivered via a helmet is currently the first-line treatment of acute pulmonary edema in most emergency departments, intensive care units and cardiology, nephrology, internal medicine, respiratory, etc. wards, while some teams even use it in the earliest stages of care in the community, in the patient's home and during transport in the ambulance.

As mentioned above, some patients with acute pulmonary edema develop a mixed acidosis in which the respiratory component appears predominant, both because of concomitant COPD and incipient fatigue of the respiratory muscles with alveolar hypoventilation and consequent hypercapnia. For this reason, ventilation with a combination of CPAP + Pressure Support (bilevel ventilation) has been and is still widely used as an alternative to CPAP. In fact, following the first negative data indicating a higher incidence of myocardial infarction in a study by Mehta et al., which was found to have some not irrelevant biases, the results of other randomized, controlled clinical trials on the use of bilevel ventilation were published. Some of these showed benefit only for hypercapnic patients, while in others the bilevel ventilation was equally effective independently of the initial carbon dioxide levels. Various meta-analyses demonstrated that, compared to oxygen therapy alone, bilevel ventilation is able to reduce the need for intubation but not survival, and that it does not increase the risk of myocardial complications, thus confirming its safety. The same studies did not reveal significant differences in various outcomes when comparing CPAP with bilevel NIV.

For the sake of correctness, we must also mention a multicenter study from England that produced partially negative results on the use of NIV in acute pulmonary edema. Both CPAP and bilevel ventilation were found to be more effective than oxygen therapy in accelerating the process of healing, but the intubation rate was not statistically significantly different between the three groups. The study raised great interest, mainly because it was published in the most important medical journal in the world, the *New England Journal of Medicine*, even though it was vitiated by many problems (e.g., very low number of intubations, <3 %; the fact that some centers were not familiar with the method of ventilation; the very advanced age of the patients) which, in our opinion, limited the scientific validity of the results.

It is a pity that this study was then used to support the choices of those who do not like NIV. However, we console ourselves with the fact that our cardiology colleagues have already included both CPAP and bilevel ventilation in their guidelines on the management of acute pulmonary edema as first-line therapy together, of course, with medical treatment. Indeed, the most recent meta-analysis, which includes the above mentioned study, confirmed the effectiveness of both NIV and CPAP in reducing the need for intubation vs standard treatment.

In conclusion, we believe that CPAP can be considered the standard treatment for acute pulmonary edema, while the bilevel mode of ventilation is to be preferred in cases characterized by marked respiratory acidosis and concomitant COPD.

11.3   Pneumonia in Immunocompromised Patients

NIV is considered the treatment of choice during episodes of acute respiratory failure in immunocompromised patients with pneumonia because of the capacity of this form of ventilation to reduce infectious complications. The presence of a focus of bronchopneumonia is relatively common in immunocompromised patients (e.g., AIDS patients, patients after chemotherapy, solid organ transplantation, or bone marrow transplantation) and, if associated with acute respiratory failure, often leads to the patient's death. The reported mortality rate of these patients when intubated and, therefore, ventilated invasively is greater than 90 %. In the 1990s, the first observational studies and case reports suggested that NIV could be a valid alternative to intubation, at the same as improving clinical outcomes. At the height of the AIDS emergency, Confalonieri and colleagues demonstrated, in a case-controlled study, that patients with *Pneumocystis carinii* pneumonia treated with NIV had a lower in-hospital mortality rate than intubated patients and also a lower rate of pneumothorax (Confalonieri et al. 2002).

Some years later, Hilbert et al., in a classical randomized study whose results were published in the *New England Journal of Medicine*, showed that early use of NIV in immunocompromised patients with lung infiltrates significantly improved gas exchange and, in particular, infectious complications, reduced the use of intubation and lowered the mortality rate compared to the same outcomes in the patients treated with standard therapy with oxygen (Hilbert et al. 2001). In detail, while the mortality rate in the NIV group was high (50 %), it was clearly lower than that in the group treated traditionally (81 %). In the wake of this study, numerous other studies confirmed the results, such that NIV, also by CPAP with a helmet, is currently common practice even outside intensive care units, for example in hematology and oncology units.

When discussing respiratory complications in immunocompromised patients, we must not forget subjects who have received a solid organ transplant. Antonelli and colleagues randomized such patients to receive NIV or standard medical therapy and oxygen (Antonelli et al. 2000). The PaO$_2$/FiO$_2$ ratio improved in 70 % of the former group and in only 25 % in the latter group, such that the use of intubation and the number of fatal complications were lower in the NIV group. The mean time spent in intensive care and the mortality rate in intensive care both decreased significantly, although in-hospital mortality did not. Given the difficulties in undertaking a study of this sort and possible medico-legal problems (particularly in the USA), this work has never been replicated since.

In conclusion, the data from this very particular population suggest that NIV should be used early to prevent intubation rather than to replace it in immunocompromised patients with acute respiratory failure.

11.4   Weaning from Invasive Ventilation in COPD

Although NIV is associated, as we have seen, with a high percentage of success in the management of exacerbations of COPD, some subjects must nevertheless be intubated for various reasons, such as a severely depressed sensorium, respiratory arrest, impossibility of removing secretions, and hemodynamic instability. If all goes well, the recourse to intubation rapidly resolves the problem that made NIV impossible to use. For example, a reduction in the PaCO$_2$ should improve the level of consciousness, just as energetic bronchial lavage, possibly associated with antibiotic treatment, could reduce the bulk of secretion and enable a new trial with NIV. Based on this physiological rationale, some uncontrolled studies suggested NIV as a method for shortening the period of intubation. In 1998, in the first randomized, controlled study, we treated one group of patients with traditional weaning through Pressure Support with the tube *in situ* and another group to early extubation (after 2–3 days) and application of NIV as a "bridge" to weaning (Nava et al. 1998). This is only possible if the patient has favorable clinical criteria, such as a reasonable degree of collaboration, sufficient capacity to expectorate, not severely altered gas exchange and a minimal ability to breathe autonomously. The method we used drastically shortened the weaning time and also had a positive effect on hospital stay and number of infectious complications, such as pneumonia, thus improving the 3-month survival rate.

Two subsequent randomized, controlled studies in France and in Brazil confirmed the concept presented above, which was also validated in another study carried out in patients who failed repeated trials of "traditional" weaning, showing that NIV, applied early after extubation, can reduce the duration of total ventilation, infectious pulmonary complications, and the time spent in an intensive care unit.

Burns et al. in a meta-analysis and systematic review identified 12 randomized controlled trials involving 530 participants, mostly with chronic obstructive pulmonary disease. Compared with invasive weaning, non invasive weaning was associated with significantly reduced mortality (relative risk 0.55, 95 % confidence interval 0.38–0.79), ventilator associated pneumonia (0.29, 95 % confidence interval 0.19–0.45),, length of stay in intensive care unit (weighted mean difference −6.27 days, −8.77 to −3.78) and hospital (−7.19 days, −10.80 to −3.58), total duration of ventilation, and duration of invasive ventilation. Non invasive weaning had no effect on weaning failures or weaning time.

More recently Girault et al. completed a randomized controlled trial in a large number of patients with chronic hypercapnic respiratory failure intubated for acute respiratory failure in 17 centers in France. Patients were randomized into three groups either to continue invasive mechanical ventilation with conventional weaning, to receive oxygen therapy after extubation, or to start NIV. Reintubation rates were 30, 37, and 32 % for the invasive weaning, oxygen-therapy and NIV groups, respectively. Weaning failure rates, including post-extubation acute respiratory failure, were 54, 71, and 33 %, respectively and this was statistically significant in favor of NIV. Rescue NIV success rates for the invasive and oxygen-therapy groups were 45 and 58 %, respectively. Apart from a longer weaning time in the NIV group than in the invasive group (2.5 vs. 1.5 days; $p = 0.033$), no significant outcome difference was observed between groups. It was therefore concluded that NIV decreases the duration of intubation and may improve the weaning results in difficult-to-wean patients with hypercapnic respiratory failure, by reducing the risk of post-extubation acute respiratory failure.

In order to convince even the most skeptical person that NIV is ventilation to all effects and not a poor relative of invasive ventilation, we conducted physiological evaluations of about 10 patients just before they were extubated and immediately after extubation when they were ventilated non invasively with the same parameters. The gas exchange and the work load of the respiratory muscles were exactly the same with the two methods of ventilation and definitely more advantageous than spontaneous breathing. This unequivocally shows that, in the stable patient, the switch from intubation to NIV merely means a change in the interface of the ventilation, but not its physiological effects. Although it cannot be used in all disorders or in all clinical settings, since it needs careful and continuous monitoring by medical and paramedical staff, we strongly believe that this method of weaning can be advantageous for some well-selected patients, above all those with COPD or chronic hypercapnia.

11.5   Prevention of Post-Extubation Respiratory Failure in High-Risk Subjects

Post-extubation respiratory failure is certainly a much more common occurrence than often thought; indeed, more than 15 % of subjects develop this complication in the 24–48 h after a weaning trial considered satisfactory. The more alarming fact is that about 40–50 % of these patients die once re-intubated. The efforts of researchers are, therefore, focused on the earliest possible treatment of patients who show initial signs of respiratory distress after being extubated. Unfortunately, as we shall see in the next chapter, waiting until the patient becomes symptomatic in some way could be too late.

Numerous epidemiological studies have identified the main causes of re-intubation, which can be summarized as the presence of comorbid conditions (in particular, chronic respiratory and cardiac disorders), upper airway problems, difficulty in expectoration, chronic hypercapnia, advanced age, and a fairly high severity score at the time of extubation. Taking into account these characteristics, three randomized controlled studies evaluated whether early application of NIV as pure prevention of possible post-extubation respiratory failure is actually able to reduce recourse to re-intubation.

The data from the first two studies were almost identical. Both studies showed that NIV administered sequentially for a few hours a day in the first 2 or 3 days after extubation in subjects who were at risk, but completely asymptomatic, significantly reduced the percentage of cases of re-intubation compared to that in patients simply kept under observation as usual practice. The studies differed only with regards to the effect on mortality, which was statistically significant in the Spanish study, whereas it just failed to be so in ours. An improvement in survival was demonstrated in a subgroup of patients who were hypercapnic at the time of extubation, confirming the fact that NIV seems to be particularly useful in the presence of high values of $PaCO_2$. This concept was recently validated in the third randomized, controlled trial carried out by the same Spanish group. All these studies excluded, *a priori*, patients with a high body weight in order to avoid factors that could confound the results. Some North American colleagues joked that since most of their patients are overweight, this indication for NIV does not have a future in the USA. Just to contradict them, a few months later it was a precisely an American study which demonstrated that preventive administration of NIV after extubation is associated, also in obese subjects, with a lower rate of re-intubation and improved survival compared with traditional behavior.

In conclusion, using NIV as a strategy to avoid the development of post-extubation respiratory failure is associated with a lower percentage of new requirement of mechanical invasive ventilation and, possibly, with improved survival.

Suggested Reading

Exacerbation of COPD

Bott J, Carroll MP, Conway JH et al (1993) Randomised controlled trial of nasal ventilation in acute ventilatory failure due to chronic obstructive airways disease. Lancet 341(8869):1555–1557

Barbé F, Togores B, Rubì M et al (1996) Noninvasive ventilatory support does not facilitate recovery from acute respiratory failure in chronic obstructive pulmonary disease. Eur Respir J 9(6):1240–1245

Brochard L, Isabey D, Piquet J et al (1990) Reversal of acute exacerbations of chronic obstructive lung disease by inspiratory assistance with a face mask. N Engl J Med 323(22):1523–1530

Brochard L, Mancebo J, Wysocki M et al (1995) Noninvasive ventilation for acute exacerbations of chronic obstructive pulmonary disease. N Engl J Med 333(13):817–822

Celikel T, Sungur M, Ceyhan B, Karakurt S (1998) Comparison of noninvasive positive ventilation with standard medical therapy in hypercapnic acute respiratory failure. Chest 114(6):1636–1642

Conti G, Antonelli M, Navalesi P et al (2002) Noninvasive vs. conventional mechanical ventilation in patients with chronic obstructive pulmonary disease after failure of medical treatment in the ward: a randomized trial. Intensive Care Med 28(12):1701–1707

Jurjevic M, Matic I, Sakic-Zdravcevic K et al (2009) Mechanical ventilation in chronic obstructive pulmonary disease patients, noninvasive vs. invasive method (randomized prospective study). Coll Antropol 33(3):791–797

Khilnani GC, Saikia N, Banga A et al (2010) Non-invasive ventilation for acute exacerbation of COPD with very high PaCO(2): a randomized controlled trial. Lung India 27(3):125–130

Keenan SP, Sinuff T, Cook DJ, Hill NS (2003) Which patients with acute exacerbation of chronic obstructive pulmonary disease benefit from noninvasive positive-pressure ventilation? A systematic review of the literature. Ann Intern Med 138(11):861–870

Plant PK, Owen JL, Elliott MW (2000) A multicentre randomised controlled trial of the early use of non-invasive ventilation in acute exacerbation of chronic obstructive pulmonary disease on general respiratory wards. Lancet 335(9219):1931–1935

Ram FS, Picot J, Lightowler J, Wedzicha JA (2004) Non-invasive positive pressure ventilation for treatment of respiratory failure due to exacerbations of chronic obstructive pulmonary disease. Cochrane Database Syst Rev (3):CD004104

Squadrone E, Frigerio P, Fogliati C et al (2004) Noninvasive vs invasive ventilation in COPD patients with severe acute respiratory failure deemed to require ventilatory assistance. Intensive Care Med 30(7):1303–1310

Acute Pulmonary Edema

Bellone A, Monari A, Cortellaro F et al (2004) Myocardial infarction rate in acute pulmonary edema: noninvasive pressure support ventilation versus continuous positive airway pressure. Crit Care Med 32(9):1860–1865

Bellone A, Vettorello M, Monari A et al (2005) Noninvasive pressure support ventilation vs. continuous positive airway pressure in acute hypercapnic pulmonary edema. Intensive Care Med 31(6):807–811

Gray A, Goodacre S, Newby DE et al (2008) Noninvasive ventilation in acute cardiogenic pulmonary edema. N Engl J Med 359(2):142–151

Mariani J, Macchia A, Belziti E et al (2011) Noninvasive ventilation in acute cardiogenic pulmonary edema: a meta-analysis of randomized controlled trials. J Cardiac Fail 17:850–859

Masip J, Betbesé AJ, Pàez J et al (2000) Non-invasive pressure support ventilation versus conventional oxygen therapy in acute cardiogenic pulmonary oedema: a randomised trial. Lancet 356(9248):26–32

Mehta S, Jay GD, Woolard RH et al (1997) Randomized, prospective trial of bilevel versus continuous positive airway pressure in acute pulmonary edema. Crit Care Med 25(4):620–628

Nava S, Carbone G, Dibattista N et al (2003) Noninvasive ventilation in cardiogenic pulmonary edema: a multicenter, randomized trial. Am J Respir Crit Care Med 168(12):1432–1437

Nouira S, Boukef R, Bouida W et al (2011) Non-invasive pressure support ventilation and CPAP in cardiogenic pulmonary edema: a multicenter randomized study in the emergency department. Intensive Care Med 37:249–256

Park M, Sangean MC, Volpe Mde S et al (2004) Randomized, prospective trial of oxygen, continuous positive airway pressure, and bilevel positive airway pressure by face mask in acute cardiogenic pulmonary edema. Crit Care Med 32(12):2407–2415

Peter JV, Moran JL, Phillips-Hughes J et al (2006) Effect of non-invasive positive pressure ventilation (NIPPV) on mortality in patients with acute cardiogenic pulmonary oedema: a meta-analysis. Lancet 367(9517):1155–1163

Immunocompromised Patients

Antonelli M, Conti G, Buffi M et al (2000) Noninvasive ventilation for treatment of acute respiratory failure in patients undergoing solid organ transplantation: a randomized trial. JAMA 283(2):235–241

Blot F, Guiguet M, Nitenberg G et al (1997) Prognostic factors for neutropenic patients in an intensive care unit: respective roles of underlying malignancies and acute organ failure. Eur J Cancer 33(7):1031–1037

Confalonieri M, Calderoni E, Terraciano S et al (2002) Noninvasive ventilation for treating acute respiratory failure in AIDS patients with Pneumocystis carinii pneumonia. Intensive Care Med 28(9):1233–1238

Hilbert G, Gruson D, Vargas F et al (2001) Noninvasive ventilation in immunosuppressed patients with pulmonary infiltrates, fever, and acute respiratory failure. N Engl J Med 344(7):481–487

Weaning Patients with COPD from Invasive Ventilation

Burns KE, Adhikari NK, Keenan SP, Meade M (2009) Use of non-invasive ventilation to wean critically ill adults off invasive ventilation: meta-analysis and systematic review. BMJ 338:1574

Ferrer M, Esquinas A, Arancibia F et al (2003) Noninvasive ventilation during persistent weaning failure: a randomized controlled trial. Am J Respir Crit Care Med 168(1):70–76

Girault C, Daudenthun I, Chevron V et al (1999) Noninvasive ventilation a systematic extubation and weaning technique in acute-on-chronic respiratory failure: a prospective, randomized controlled study. Am J Respir Crit Care Med 160(1):86–92

Girault C, Bubenheim M, Abroug F. et al for the VENISE trial group (2011) Noninvasive ventilation and weaning in patients with chronic hypercapnic respiratory failure. A randomized multicenter trial. Am J Respir Crit Care Med 184: 672–679

Nava S, Ambrosino N, Clini E et al (1998) Noninvasive mechanical ventilation in the weaning of patients with respiratory failure due to chronic obstructive pulmonary disease. A randomized, controlled trial. Ann Intern Med 128(9):721–728

Trevisan CE, Vieira SR (2008) Noninvasive mechanical ventilation may be useful in treating patients who fail weaning from invasive mechanical ventilation: a randomized clinical trial. Crit Care 12(2):R51

Prevention of Post-Extubation Respiratory Failure in Patients at Risk

Epstein SK, Ciubotaru RL, Wong JB (1997) Effect of failed extubation on the outcome of mechanical ventilation. Chest 112(1):186–192

El Solh AA, Aquilina A, Pineda L et al (2006) Noninvasive ventilation for prevention of postextubation respiratory failure in obese patients. Eur Respir J 28(3):588–595

Ferrer M, Valencia M, Nicolas JM et al (2006) Early noninvasive ventilation averts extubation failure in patients at risk: a randomized trial. Am J Respir Crit Care Med 173(2):164–170

Ferrer M, Sellarés J, Valencia M et al (2009) Non-invasive ventilation after extubation in hypercapnic patients with chronic respiratory disorders: randomised controlled trial. Lancet 374:1082–1088

Nava S, Gregoretti C, Fanfulla F et al (2005) Noninvasive ventilation to prevent respiratory failure after extubation in high-risk patients. Crit Care Med 33(11):2465–2470

NIV in the Treatment of Acute Respiratory Failure: Emerging Indications

12

12.1 Prevention and Treatment of Surgical Complications

This is definitely an emerging field of application. It has been known for some time now that the period following thoracic surgery and major abdominal surgery can be complicated by hypoxia. This is almost always related to poor mobility of the diaphragm, which can be the consequence of traumatic damage during the operation, a pharmacological effect of the anesthetics and/or analgesics on the phrenic nerve or more banally the intense pain that prevents the patient from expanding the respiratory system adequately (i.e. the chest cage and abdomen). Decreased diaphragmatic function is associated with reduced pulmonary compliance and areas of atelectasia, which are the main risk factors for the development of pneumonia. This much feared complication of the post-operative period can, in some cases, be fatal.

For example, the development of hypoxia following respiratory complications in patients undergoing pneumectomy or lobectomy is associated with an approximately 50 % mortality rate. The prevention of atelectasia has, therefore, always been one of the aims of post-operative rehabilitation. Already in the 1980s, it was thought that the application of a positive pressure through a CPAP mask would be able to reduce the work of the respiratory muscles and on the other hand promote early recruitment of poorly aerated regions of the lungs. The first, pioneering studies, regarding both abdominal and thoracic surgery, demonstrated that following X-ray evidence of post-operative atelectasia, it was possible to reduce or prevent pneumonia and loss of respiratory function (in terms of volume) and improve gas exchange. More recently, some researchers have focused on the prevention of respiratory complications starting treatment even before the operation or immediately after the surgical procedure has been completed. Two randomized controlled trials are particularly interesting. Auriant and colleagues demonstrated that the early use of NIV to treat incipient respiratory failure after pulmonary resection was not only able to reduce the need for intubation, but even improved survival (Auriant et al. 2001). In a multicenter trial carried out in Piedmont (Italy), Squadrone and colleagues showed how the application of CPAP through a helmet significantly reduced the incidences of intubation, pneumonia

S. Nava and F. Fanfulla, *Non Invasive Artificial Ventilation*,
DOI: 10.1007/978-88-470-5526-1_12, © Springer-Verlag Italia 2014

and septic complications (Squadrone et al. 2005). This use of a helmet is very interesting since such patients often receive their treatment outside an intensive care unit, where ease of use is a fundamental determinant of acceptance by staff.

In conclusion, although the evidence has not reached level 1, predominantly because of the different techniques of ventilation used (NIV and CPAP) and the different clinical scenarios (thoracic and abdominal surgery), we feel that we can state that the most immediate new frontier of use of NIV is the post-operative setting.

12.2   Obesity Hypoventilation Syndrome

As we know well, obesity is becoming a serious socioeconomic problem, as well as a public health problem of primary importance.

This pathological state predisposes some patients to chronic alveolar hypoventilation, in some cases associated with obstructive apnea syndrome. In the light of what has already been stated, this would be an ideal field for the use of NIV and yet, surprisingly, there are very few studies to date on the use of NIV in this form of respiratory failure and most of the ones that have been done are observational studies. These studies confirm what we all expected, that is, a reduction in recourse to intubation and an improvement in blood gases.

Personally, we believe that at least a "judicious" careful attempt should be made in these conditions, although being aware that if intubation is needed in these patients, it could be difficult. Furthermore, perhaps the time has come to organize a multicenter, randomized trial to establish scientifically the role of NIV in obesity hypoventilation syndrome.

12.3   Palliation of Symptoms in the Terminally Ill Patient

The real title of this section should be "palliation and treatment of the patient who refuses intubation." Unfortunately in Italy, it is still impossible to discuss expected directives in a constructive, serious manner, as has been done in almost all civilized countries, with the result that it is still a taboo to tackle this problem. The sensation is that everything is left hypocritically in the hands of healthcare staff so that, with a paternalistic spirit or sometimes with cynicism, we decide what is good and what is not good to do.

That said, there are numerous publications on the use of NIV in patients who have reached the terminal stage of their illness and whose life expectancy is, by definition, very short and in whom pharmacological treatment has reached the so-called ceiling without providing additional benefits. These patients are rarely, if ever, admitted to an intensive care unit because of the known bed shortage and reach our attention exhausted by dyspnea and with a respiratory distress that has become insupportable.

The first thing to do is to ask yourself whether this deterioration is reversible or not. Three observational studies have demonstrated that the use of NIV in patients with acute respiratory failure who have decided not to be intubated is more effective in the case of an exacerbation of COPD or acute heart failure than in other conditions such as tumors or pneumonia. Indeed, about half of the patients with the former two causes of respiratory failure can be discharged from hospital compared with 15–20 % of other patients, particularly those with cancer.

Our survey, sponsored by the European Respiratory Society, confirmed that also in the real world of subintensive care units, the use of NIV as the "last" treatment (or 'ceiling NIV') is fairly popular given that about 30 % of the patients admitted into these structures in a terminal stage of their chronic respiratory disease receive this treatment.

The major problem, also from an ethical point of view, is to understand how closely this method approaches futile medical care, prolonging a patient's suffering once the acute event has been resolved, or how much it extends an existence that appears acceptable and is accepted by the patient. Here there is a difficult concept to measure, particularly in these conditions: the quality of remaining life. This is not easily quantifiable by either questionnaires or scales. For example, when two patients were asked why they insisted on being kept alive, one answered "because I want to see my first grandchild, who will be born in 2 months" while the other needed 3 months to see his favorite football team finally win the national league. While we might all be able to understand the former, even fans of the same football team might find it more difficult to understand the latter! Nevertheless, a person's wishes should always be respected.

NIV could be considered the more natural and less traumatic support in this difficult period of a person's life, given that its suspension would be less cruel than, for example, extubation. A particular case is when dyspnea occurs suddenly in the terminal stage of a patient's disease. Although numerous studies have demonstrated that it not at all easy to predict the real survival of patients, we are often faced with patients with insupportable dyspnea (or rather, pain of the respiratory system), in the last hours of their life. A classical example is a patient affected by a solid tumor or one with a malignancy of the hematopoietic system. A search of the literature would surprise you, because there are no studies demonstrating the efficacy of oxygen in reducing dyspnea and, therefore, the last resort is morphine, although this could dull the senses of the patient who perhaps wants to stay lucid to say goodbye to his dear ones or deal with last bureaucratic business. A pilot study in patients with solid tumors showed that in a good percentage of cases (about 60 %) the use of NIV was able to reduce dyspnea.

The first randomized, controlled multicenter study designed to determine the feasibility and effects of NIV versus oxygen on dyspnea in patients with end-stage cancer and respiratory distress showed that NIV is more effective than oxygen in reducing dyspnoea and decreasing the doses of morphine needed in patients with end-stage cancer. However, also in these circumstances, we should evaluate each case individually to ensure that we do not indiscriminately prolong a patient's suffering.

In conclusion, in such a delicate, but emerging field, NIV appears to be an additional instrument for improving, as much as possible, the quality of death but certainly not that of life, which it is futile to try to do at this stage.

12.4   Asthma

This is a relatively unexplored and controversial field of application of NIV. Observational studies have shown that NIV can be a valid alternative to intubation even when a patient has become hypercapnic. We have used the words "even when" because during the initial stages of an asthma attack, the patient tries to compensate for the unpleasant sensation caused by the bronchial obstruction by increasing his or her minute ventilation, that is, by hyperventilating. The development of hypercapnia is prognostically a very worrying sign since it means that the respiratory pump is failing and that the patient's conditions are worsening rapidly. In the absence of randomized controlled trials or more robust studies, we do not feel that we can recommend the use of NIV in the presence of a high $PaCO_2$.

On the other hand, the situation is different when the ventilation method is used to prevent a possible worsening of the patient's conditions. Two controlled studies have been carried out in patients without frank respiratory failure, comparing the effect of NIV and placebo ventilation. In one study NIV improved peak inspiratory flow and in the other it decreased hospital admissions. The effects described in the former of the two studies could only be achieved with high insufflation pressures and not with low ones or medical therapy alone. An important detail, described later, is that bronchodilator therapy can be administered during NIV and so ventilatory support does not need to be suspended in order to give drugs.

Thus, the current rationale for the use of NIV during an attack of asthma is only that of preventing further worsening, but not as a real treatment of the respiratory failure. Nevertheless, in a protected environment, a brief trial of NIV can also be indicated in a patient in a critical condition.

12.5   Restrictive Neuromuscular and Chest Cage Disorders

It is really surprising that we all seem to have successfully ventilated at least one patient of this type in our career and yet there are so few studies on the issue.

I remember the first patient in whom I (S.N.) used NIV for the very first time in my life was a woman with kyphoscoliosis and very severe hypercapnic respiratory failure. The success achieved not only astonished me, but also my colleagues at that time, and it was perhaps then that my enthusiasm for NIV was born.

Having said this, there is a common belief that the main application of NIV is restrictive disorders and that this form of ventilation works better in these disorders than in COPD. However, the only study that has analyzed this problem showed the reverse: NIV was more effective at reducing the need for intubation in patients with exacerbation of COPD than in patients with hypercapnia caused by other restrictive chest disorders.

The only study, performed in Italy, which has compared NIV versus invasive ventilation in a small group of patients with neuromuscular diseases showed a series of improvements in clinical outcomes in the group ventilated non invasively. In fairness it should be said that the patients in the group treated NIV did have mini-tracheotomies to enable efficient removal of bronchial secretions, so the method should be considered "partially" non invasive.

In conclusion, despite the fact that clinical experience suggests that restrictive diseases respond well to the application of NIV, we are still waiting for firm scientific evidence.

12.6   Ventilatory Support During Bronchoscopy

This use of NIV in bronchoscopy was described more than a decade ago in a study performed by Prof. Antonelli's group in Rome (Antonelli et al. 2002). It is still common practice to use preventive intubation in severely hypoxic patients before carrying out fibrobronchoscopy. We are thinking, for example, about patients with severe pneumonia or an exacerbation of pulmonary fibrosis in whom we must carry out at least bronchoalveolar lavage and/or transbronchial biopsy. By taking due precautions, maintaining careful monitoring and, above all, having appropriate equipment available (i. e., good CPAP or a good ventilator and particularly a mask with an *ad hoc* and not self-made orifice), these interventions can be carried out safely, even in very hypoxic patients, without necessarily having to use more invasive measures (Fig. 12.1). Randomized studies against high-flow oxygen have demonstrated the efficacy of NIV or CPAP (for example with the Boussignac system) in drastically reducing desaturations both during and after the interventions. A more recent observational study also demonstrated that bronchoscopy could be performed in patients using a helmet as the ventilator interface. For curiosity's sake, we also mention a study by Natalini et al. who used external negative pressure ventilation to carry out bronchoscopy using a rigid instrument (Natalini et al. 1998).

In conclusion, this is a rapidly expanding application which should, in our opinion, become a first-line procedure in hypoxic patients who must undergo diagnostic bronchoscopy.

12.7   Future Indications Supported by Single Studies

In this paragraph, we briefly mention some potential applications of NIV which have so far only been supported by single observational studies and precisely for this reason, although interesting, require further confirmation.

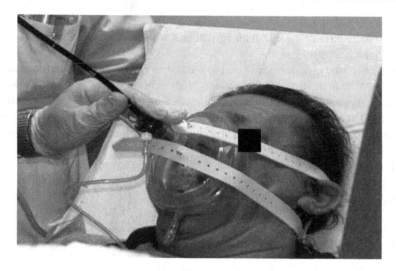

Fig. 12.1 Bronchoscopy made possible by NIV in a severely hypoxic patient

For example, NIV has been used to treat acute respiratory failure secondary to disorders such as exacerbations of cystic fibrosis, pulmonary fibrosis, thoracic trauma with flail chest, acute pancreatitis, or as a bridge in patients who are to be transplanted or in whom intubation could be a limit to the indication for the intervention.

Suggested Reading

Prevention and Treatment of Surgical Complications

Auriant I, Jallot A, Hervé P et al (2001) Noninvasive ventilation reduces mortality in acute respiratory failure following lung resection. Am J Respir Crit Care Med 164(7):1231–1235

Chiumello D, Chevallard G, Gregoretti C (2011) Non-invasive ventilation in postoperative patients: a systematic review. Intensive Care Med 37:918–929

Joris JL, Sottiaux TM, Chiche JD et al (1997) Effect of bi-level positive airway pressure (BiPAP) nasal ventilation on the postoperative pulmonary restrictive syndrome in obese patients undergoing gastroplasty. Chest 111(3):665–670

Kutlu CA, Williams EA, Evans TW et al (2000) Acute lung injury and acute respiratory distress syndrome after pulmonary resection. Ann Thorac Surg 69(2):376–380

Perrin C, Jullien V, Vénissac N et al (2007) Prophylactic use of noninvasive ventilation in patients undergoing lung resectional surgery. Respir Med 101(7):1572–1578

Pinilla JC, Oleniuk FH, Tan L et al (1990) Use of nasal continuous positive airway pressure mask in the treatment of postoperative atelectasis in aortocoronary bypass surgery. Crit Care Med 18(8):836–840

Squadrone V, Coha M, Cerutti E et al (2005) Continuous positive airway pressure for treatment of postoperative hypoxemia: a randomized controlled trial. JAMA 293(5):589–595

Obesity Hypoventilation Syndrome

Nelson JA, Loredo JS, Acosta JA (2011) The obesity-hypoventilation syndrome and respiratory failure in the acute trauma patient. J Emerg Med 40(4):e67–e69

Pérez de Llano LA, Golpe R, Ortiz Piquer M et al (2005) Short-term and long-term effects of nasal intermittent positive pressure ventilation in patients with obesity-hypoventilation syndrome. Chest 128(2):587–594

Palliation of Symptoms in Terminally Ill Patients

Azoulay E, Demoule A, Jaber S et al (2011) Palliative noninvasive ventilation in patients with acute respiratory failure. Intensive Care Med 37:1250–1257

Azoulay E, Kouatchet A, Jaber S et al (2013) Noninvasive mechanical ventilation in patients having declined tracheal intubation. Intensive Care Med 39:292–301

Cuomo A, Delmastro M, Ceriana P et al (2004) Noninvasive mechanical ventilation as a palliative treatment of acute respiratory failure in patients with end-stage solid cancer. Palliat Med 18(7):602–610

Curtis JR, Cook DJ, Sinuff T et al (2007) Noninvasive positive pressure ventilation in critical and palliative care settings: understanding the goals of therapy. Crit Care Med 35(3):932–939

Fernandez R, Baigorri F, Artigas A (2007) Noninvasive ventilation in patients with "do-not-intubate" orders: medium-term efficacy depends critically on patient selection. Intensive Care Med 33(2):350–354

Levy M, Tanios MA, Nelson D et al (2004) Outcomes of patients with do-not-intubate orders treated with noninvasive ventilation. Crit Care Med 32(10):2002–2007

Nava S, Sturani C, Hartl S et al (2007) End-of-life decision-making in respiratory intermediate care units: a European survey. Eur Respir J 30(1):156–164

Nava S, Ferrer M, Esquinas A et al (2013) Palliative use of non-invasive ventilation in end-of-life patients with solid tumours: a randomised feasibility trial. Lancet Oncol 14:219–227

Prinicipi T, Pantanetti S, Catani F et al (2004) Noninvasive continuous positive airway pressure delivered by helmet in hematological malignancy patients with hypoxemic acute respiratory failure. Intensive Care Med 30(1):147–150

Schettino G, Altobelli N, Kocmarek RM (2005) Noninvasive positive pressure ventilation reverses acute respiratory failure in selected "do-not-intubate" patients. Crit Care Med 33:1976–1982

Asthma

Soma T, Hino M, kida K, Kudoh S (2008) A Prospective and randomized study for improvement of acute asthma by non-invasive positive pressure ventilation (NPPV). Intern Med 47(6):493–501

Soroksky A, Stav D, Shpirer I (2003) A pilot, prospective, randomized, placebo-controlled trial of bilevel positive airway pressure in acute asthmatic attack. Chest 123(4):1018–1025

Restrictive Neuromuscular and Chest Cage Disorders

Puha J, Kong K, Lee KH et al (2005) Noninvasive ventilation in hypercapnic acute respiratory
    failure due to chronic obstructive pulmonary disease vs. other conditions: effectiveness and
    predictors of failure. Intensive Care Med 31(4):533–539
Vianello A, Bevilacqua M, Arcaro G et al (2000) Non-invasive ventilatory approach to treatment
    of acute respiratory failure in neuromuscular disorders. A comparison with endotracheal
    intubation. Intensive Care Med 26(4):384–390

Ventilatory Support During Bronchoscopy

Antonelli M, Conti G, Rocco M et al (2002) Noninvasive positive-pressure ventilation versus
    conventional oxygen supplementation in hypoxemic patients undergoing diagnostic bron-
    choscopy. Chest 121(4):1149–1154
Antonelli M, Pennisi MA, Conti G et al (2003) Fiberoptic bronchoscopy during noninvasive
    positive pressure ventilation delivered by helmet. Intensive Care Med 29(1):126–129
Maitre B, Jaber S, Maggiore SM et al (2000) Continuous positive airway pressure during
    fiberoptic bronchoscopy in hypoxemic patients. A randomized double-blind study using a new
    device. Am J Respir Crit Care Med 162(3 Pt 1):1063–1067
Natalini G, Cavaliere S, Vitacca M et al (1998) Negative pressure ventilation vs. spontaneous
    assisted ventilation during rigid bronchoscopy. A controlled randomised trial. Acta
    Anaesthesiol Scand 42(9):1063–1069

Future Indications Supported by Single Studies

Ambrosino N, Guarracino F (2011) Unusual applications of noninvasive ventilation. Eur Respir J
    38:440–449
Yokoyama T, Kondoh Y, Taniguchi H et al (2010) Noninvasive ventilation in acute exacerbation
    of idiopathic pulmonary fibrosis. Inter Med 49:1509–1514
Jaber S, Chanques G, Sebbane M et al (2006) Noninvasive positive pressure ventilation in
    patients with respiratory failure due to severe acute pancreatitis. Respiration 73(2):166–172
Mollica C, Paone G, Conti V et al (2010) Mechanical ventilation in patients with end-stage
    idiopathic pulmonary fibrosis. Respiration 79:209–215
O'Brien G, Criner GJ (1999) Mechanical ventilation as a bridge to lung transplantation. J Heart
    Lung Transplant 18(3):255–265
Smyth A (2006) Update on treatment of pulmonary exacerbations in cystic fibrosis. Curr Opin
    Pulm Med 12(6):440–444
Xirouchaki N, Kondoudaki E, Anastasaki M (2005) Noninvasive bilevel positive pressure
    ventilation in patients with blunt thoracic trauma. Respiration 72(5):517–522

NIV in the Treatment of Acute Respiratory Failure: Controversial Indications

13

13.1 Pneumonia

A case of pneumonia that requires ventilation, whether invasively or non invasively, is always a serious event associated with a high mortality rate, particularly in the elderly, even though it is often considered by the media as an infection that is "easy" to resolve.

Why is this a controversial indication for NIV? Because there are observational studies that are absolutely against the use of NIV and a couple of randomized controlled trial in favor, in theory, but not necessarily in all cases of pneumonia or in all patients.

The difficulty in taking a position on this indication derives from the fact that it is not easy to compare the studies which, besides anything else, used the NIV in patients with differing severity of disease, based on the PaO_2/FiO_2 ratio. Once again it is important to talk about the timing of application. Nobody would consider intubating a patient with a PaO_2/FiO_2 between 250 and 300, although it is precisely in this category of patient that NIV could act best as prevention to avoid a subsequent worsening. This concept is supported by Cosentini et al. (2010) who used this philosophy in the treatment of patients with pneumonia, ventilating the patients with CPAP through a helmet in the Accident and Emergency department. CPAP delivered by helmet rapidly improved oxygenation in patients with community-acquired pneumonia suffering from a moderate hypoxemic acute respiratory failure. This trial represents a proof-of-concept evaluation of the potential usefulness of CPAP in patients with community-acquired pneumonia.

The data are much less encouraging when NIV is used as a true alternative to intubation. On this subject we advise you to read the article by Domenighetti, a Ticinese friend who, breaking out of the typical framework of evidence-based medicine, has launched a very important clinical message: for equivalent levels of hypoxia, patients with acute pulmonary edema have a clearly better outcome than those with pneumonia, despite the initial improvement in blood-gases (Domenighetti et al. 2002).

S. Nava and F. Fanfulla, *Non Invasive Artificial Ventilation*,
DOI: 10.1007/978-88-470-5526-1_13, © Springer-Verlag Italia 2014

In other words, the PaO_2/FiO_2 ratio is important, but it is also an umbrella under which we group different disorders with different pathophysiological backgrounds and times of onset; it is not, therefore, surprising that we also observe completely different responses to NIV. Of course, this not only applies to acute pulmonary edema and pneumonias, but to all those disorders that lead to hypoxia.

The randomized controlled trial to which we referred early is that by Confalonieri and colleagues, who compared NIV versus standard medical therapy + oxygen (Confalonieri et al. 1999). Overall, the results were in favor of NIV, in that significantly fewer of the patients in the group treated this way required intubation. However, a post hoc analysis showed that this was entirely due to the subgroup of patients with COPD and hypercapnia on admission. A high $PaCO_2$ is, therefore, the *leit-motif* for obtaining favorable results.

In conclusion, the advice is to use NIV as early as possible in patients with pneumonia, remembering that it is the hypercapnic patient who is the ideal candidate and that applying NIV could lead to disappointing results not only for you but above all for your patients.

13.2 Acute Respiratory Distress Syndrome

The mortality rate of patients with acute respiratory distress syndrome (ARDS) is very high and even now it still reaches 30–40 %. We are, therefore, talking about a disorder that should always be treated in an intensive care unit except, perhaps, for the earliest stages but in any case in a protected environment. We should also say that, for reasons of safety, any trial with NIV should only be performed in the absence of multiorgan failure and in patients who are hemodynamically stable, without sepsis and never with a PaO_2/FiO_2 below 150.

For example, a randomized study by Ferrer et al., carried out in patients with hypoxic respiratory failure, demonstrated the efficacy of NIV versus standard therapy in reducing recourse to intubation but, at the same time, showed that the patients with the highest risk of failure were precisely those with ARDS (Ferrer et al. 2003). A review of the literature leads us to be very prudent concerning the use of NIV. One study always reported as a "positive" one was published in the *New England Journal of Medicine* by Antonelli and colleagues, who demonstrated that an improvement in oxygenation 1 h after starting treatment could be obtained by using either traditional intubation or NIV, with the latter being associated with a significant reduction in severe complications (Antonelli et al. 1998). The study by Antonelli is certainly robust and well designed and has, therefore, become one of the most frequently cited works in the literature; nevertheless, due care should be taken before generalizing its results. First of all, the study is often referred to as having been carried out in patients with ARDS, whereas only about 25 % of the population studied had this syndrome; furthermore, the study was performed in a single center in a hospital in which the team was particularly experienced in and enthusiastic about NIV, limiting the certainty that the results could be reproduced in every intensive care unit. A Chinese study (Zhan et al. 2012) is probably the first randomized controlled trial comparing NIV versus high-concentration oxygen in patients with mild ARDS, according to the new Berlin definition (i.e., those patients with a PaO_2/FiO_2 ratio $> 200 < 300$). A total of 21 patients were assigned to NIV and 19 to the control group. The proportion of patients requiring intubation was lower in the former group, and there was also a tendency to reduced mortality in this group.

However, a series of observational studies carried out in 'real life' situations dampened the optimism somewhat, highlighting the difficulty in treating a patient with averagely severe ARDS with NIV. A multicenter study carried out in three intensive care units with great experience in NIV is particularly interesting: this study demonstrated that, after having excluded a series of patients with hemodynamic instability, those requiring protection of the airways, and patients with severe sensorial disorders or multiorgan failure, it was possible to use NIV in about 65 % of the patient admitted to hospital. Of these cases just under a half had to be intubated subsequently because of a poor response to NIV. These patients were characterized by being male, being older, and having a higher SAPS II score (i. e. >34) and more marked hypoxia on admission (i. e. $PaO_2/FiO_2 < 175$). The development of sepsis after starting NIV was associated with a low success rate. So, if we calculate the percentage of patients in whom we can use NIV successfully in real life conditions, this is <20 %, eroding the enthusiasm of even the most optimistic individuals.

In conclusion, it is probably reasonable to use NIV for an initial, short trial period in a patient with ARDS who is hemodynamically stable and has moderate hypoxia ($PaO_2/FiO_2 > 180$), but you must be ready to intubate the patient quickly.

13.3   Treatment of Post-extubation Respiratory Failure

We are really sorry to define this indication as "controversial" since we are convinced that at least in a limited number of patients NIV has a role and a rationale. Post-extubation respiratory failure is associated with a very high mortality rate and so its treatment with non invasive strategies could, in theory, reduce at least the possible infectious complications due to intubation, which are major causes of death.

We said previously that early identification of patients at risk and preventive use of NIV for a few days is associated with a better clinical outcome, but it is not always possible to "allow" this approach for reasons of time, staff, availability of beds, and appropriate instruments. So, we often find ourselves in the intensive care unit with a patient who is progressively developing first respiratory distress and then frank respiratory failure hours after being extubated.

However, two randomized controlled trials have "demolished" the use of NIV. A multicenter, international study by Esteban et al. demonstrated that, compared to the more conservative medical therapy, in this setting NIV is associated with a higher mortality rate, probably because too long a time passes between the development of the respiratory distress and the intubation (Esteban et al. 2004). However, once again, a series of problems related to the study should be pointed out, starting with the limited experience that most of the centers involved had with NIV and finishing with the strange results obtained in the control group in which NIV could be used as rescue therapy. The success rate of NIV was greater than 50 % in this subgroup of patients, who were theoretically more severely ill, since they had already failed a trial of medical therapy, than in the group in whom NIV was used immediately.

In contrast, the other single-center study by Keenan et al. did not show any statistically significant differences in the main outcomes (i.e., re-intubation, mortality, duration of hospital admission) between patients managed with medical therapy or NIV. However, this study excluded, *a priori*, a group of patients who would theoretically have benefited most from NIV, that is, hypercapnic patients with COPD (Keenan et al. 2002). In fact, the preceding study carried out in France had shown that, compared to the effect of traditional treatment in a control group, NIV significantly reduced recourse to re-intubation precisely in the patients with post-extubation hypercapnic respiratory failure.

In conclusion, although the data from the two largest randomized controlled trials were negative, we do not feel that we can totally condemn the use of NIV in the treatment of post-extubation respiratory distress; indeed, we feel we can recommend its cautious use in patients with COPD who are hypercapnic.

13.4 Severe Acute Respiratory Syndrome and Other Pandemics

We should say immediately that the Canadian medical authorities have vetoed the use of NIV in severe acute respiratory syndrome (SARS) and the American authorities are considering this indication with considerable skepticism. We all hope that the alarm created by these pandemics is unjustified and the day of the apocalypse will never come, but let us consider that it will. Someone is going to have to explain to us where all the hundreds, if not thousands, of patients will be treated. The number of beds in intensive therapy units would clearly be insufficient, as would the availability of the more technologically advanced ventilators; furthermore, intubation is usually performed after sedation and neuromuscular blockade, which can only be done by specialists. We will, therefore, be asked to make dramatic choices between who does or does not "deserve" treatment. Perhaps, after all, we should think about alternative strategies, such as NIV, for the people who are still not very seriously ill and who could even be treated outside intensive care units.

This is not a completely unrealistic hypothesis because it is actually supported by some observational studies carried out in China during the outbreak of SARS. These studies demonstrated the efficacy, but above all the safety and feasibility, of NIV in this situation. In particular, one of these studies showed that of more than

100 healthcare workers who had been involved in using NIV, none had developed the disease or become positive for the coronavirus. Of course, all this was obtained by taking the right precautions such as admitting the patients to negative pressure rooms, and supplying the workers with special protective overalls and helmets. We should point out that not using these safety measures could put both the staff and patients at a real risk of infection since aerosol particles are sprayed for almost a meter during the phase of expiration of NIV.

This has, however, been recently challenged by Simonds et al. who showed how NIV is a droplet-generating procedure, producing droplets >10 μm, so that they are not likely to remain airborne. A few observational studies have described the outcomes of ventilated patients during the recent H1N1 pandemics, in which only a minimal part of the subjects received NIV. Most of the large multicenter studies reported moderate ($\sim$50 %) rates of NIV failure while other single center investigations have recently described a better outcome, suggesting that individual training and experience with NIV may be determinants of success in this high-risk condition.

In conclusion, we believe that NIV could be a valid alternative to intubation during a pandemic, particularly if used outside an intensive care unit. Obviously, we hope that our belief never needs to be put to the test.

Suggested Reading

Pneumonia

Confalonieri M, Potena A, Carbone G et al (1999) Acute respiratory failure in patients with severe community-acquired pneumonia. A prospective randomized evaluation of noninvasive ventilation. Am J Respir Crit Care Med 160(5 Pt 1):1585–1591

Cosentini R, Brambilla AM, Aliberti S et al (2010) Helmet CPAP versus oxygen therapy to improve oxygenation in community-acquired pneumonia: a randomized controlled trial. Chest 138:114–120

Domenighetti G, Gayer R, Gentilini R (2002) Noninvasive pressure support ventilation in non-COPD patients with acute cardiogenic pulmonary edema and severe community-acquired pneumonia: acute effects and outcome. Intensive Care Med 28(9):1226–1232

Acute Respiratory Distress Syndrome and Acute Lung Injury

Antonelli M, Conti G, Rocco M et al (1998) A comparison of noninvasive positive-pressure ventilation and conventional mechanical ventilation in patients with acute respiratory failure. N Engl J Med 339(7):429–435

Ferrer M, Esquinas A, Leon M et al (2003) Noninvasive ventilation in severe hypoxemic respiratory failure: a randomized clinical trial. Am J Respir Crit Care Med 168(12):1438–1444

Jolliet P, Abajo B, Pasquina P, Chevrolet JC (2001) Non-invasive pressure support ventilation in severe community-acquiredpneumonia. Intensive Care Med 27(5):812–821

Martin TJ, Hovis JD, Costantino JP et al (2000) A randomized, prospective evaluation of noninvasive ventilation for acute respiratory failure. Am J Respir Crit Care Med 161(3 Pt 1):807–813

Rana S, Jenad H, Gay PC et al (2006) Failure of non-invasive ventilation in patients with acute lung injury: observational cohort study. Crit Care 10(3):R79

Wysocki M, Tric L, Wolff MA (1995) Noninvasive pressure support ventilation in patients with acute respiratory failure. A randomized comparison with conventional therapy. Chest 107(3):761–768

Zhan Q, Sun B, Liang L et al (2012) Early use of noninvasive positive pressure ventilation for acute lung injury: a multicenter randomized controlled trial. Crit Care Med 4(2):455–460

Zhu Q, Sun B, Liang L et al (2012) Early use of noninvasive pressure support ventilation for acute lung injury: a multicenter randomized trial. Crit Care Med 40:455–460

Treatment of Post-extubation Respiratory Failure

Hilbert G, Gruson D, Portel L et al (1998) Noninvasive pressure support ventilation in COPD patients with postextubation hypercapnic respiratory insufficiency. Eur Respir J 11(6):1349–1353

Keenan SP, Powers C, McCormack DG, Block G (2002) Noninvasive positive-pressure ventilation for postextubation respiratory distress: a randomized controlled trial. JAMA 287(24):3238–3244

Esteban A, Frutos-Vivar F, Ferguson ND et al (2004) Noninvasive positive-pressure ventilation for respiratory failure after extubation. N Engl J Med 350(24):2452–2460

Jiang JS, Kao SJ, Wang SN (1999) Effect of early application of biphasic positive airway pressure on the outcome of extubation in ventilator weaning. Respirology 4(2):161–165

Severe Acute Respiratory Syndrome and Other Pandemics

Cheung TM, Yam LY, So LK et al (2004) Effectiveness of noninvasive positive pressure ventilation in the treatment of acute respiratory failure in severe acute respiratory syndrome. Chest 126(3):845–850

Estenssoro E, Rios FG, Apezteguia C (2010) Pandemic 2009 influenza A in Argentina: a study of 337 patients on mechanical ventilation. Am J Resp Crit Care Med 182:41–48

Han F, Jiang YY, Zheng JH et al (2004) Noninvasive positive pressure ventilation treatment for acute respiratory failure in SARS. Sleep Breath 8(2):97–106

Hui DS, Chow BK, Ng SS et al (2009) Exhaled air dispersion distances during noninvasive ventilation via different Respironics face masks. Chest 136(4):998–1005

Kumar A, Zarychanski R, Pinto R, Cook DJ, Marshall J, Lacroix J et al (2009) Critically ill patients with 2009 influenza A (H1N1) infection in Canada. JAMA 302:1872–1879

Li H, Ma RC (2010) Clinical analysis of 75 patients with severe influenza A H1N1 in Qinghai Province. Zhon W Zhon Bing J J Yi Xue 22:164–165

Nicolini A, Tonveronachi E, Navalesi P et al (2012) Effectiveness and predictors of success of noninvasive ventilation during H1N1 pandemics: a multicenter study. Minerva Anestesiol 78(12):1333–1340

Poutanen SM, Low DE, Henry B et al (2003) Identification of severe acute respiratory syndrome in Canada. N Engl J Med 348(20):1195–2005

Simonds AK, Hanak A, Chatwin M, Morrell M, Hall A et al (2010) Evaluation of droplet dispersion during non-invasive ventilation, oxygen therapy, nebuliser treatment and chest physiotherapy in clinical practice: implications for management of pandemic influenza and other airborne infections. Health Technol Assess 14:131–172

Teke T, Coskun R, Sungur M, Guven M, Bekci TT, Maden E et al (2011) 2009 H1n1 influenza and experience in three critical care units. Int J Med Sci 8:270–277

Zhan Q, Sun B, Liang L, Yan X, Zhang L, Yang J, Wang L, Ma Z, Shi L, Wei L, Li G, Yang L, Shi Z, Chen Y, Xu Q, Li W, Zhu X, Wang Z, Sun Y, Zhuo J, Liu Y, Li X, Wang C (2012) Early use of noninvasive positive pressure ventilation for acute lung injury: a multicenter randomized controlled trial. Crit Care Med 40(2):455–460. doi:10.1097/CCM.0b013e318232d75e

Zhao Z, Zhang F, Xu M et al (2003) Description and clinical treatment of an early outbreak of severe acute respiratory syndrome (SARS) in Guangzhou, PR China. J Med Microbiol 52(Pt 8):715–720

Eight Rules to Remember When Ventilating a Patient Non Invasively

14

14.1 Everything Must be Ready and Everything Must be Familiar

There must always be a ventilator ready and an emergency trolley equipped in the intensive care unit. The first rule for anyone planning to work in an emergency is to prepare the trolley with a ventilator with its tubing already attached, any non-rebreathing devices that might be used, and the highest number of interfaces possible. Having to assemble everything in a rush is a source of error and creates a frenetic sensation that right from the start will undermine trust between you and the paramedical staff, but worse still, between you and the patient. Our advice is to keep the trolley in a safe place that everyone knows and to have a check-list of items that should be on it so that they can be replaced after the trolley has been used and controlled during periodic checks by the staff. However, the fact that everything is in place does not relieve us from the duty of asking ourselves whether we know exactly how the devices that we will use work.

For example, are we sure that we remember what to do if we use a non-breathing device with dispersion holes? Do we remember where to put the PEEP on the helmet if we want to change it to increase the level of expiratory pressure? We are using life-saving devices and we cannot allow ourselves the indulgence of learning by "trial and error," the approach that we now use when faced with a new mobile phone or other electronic device. If you are folding a parachute you must know what you are doing, particularly if you are folding your own!

14.2 There is No Such Thing as the Best Method of Ventilation

As seen previously, there are many techniques for NIV, none of which has been demonstrated to be clearly superior to the others in the treatment of acute respiratory failure. Patients have individual and unpredictable responses and so the common practice is to use the ventilator and the method that enables the

S. Nava and F. Fanfulla, *Non Invasive Artificial Ventilation*,
DOI: 10.1007/978-88-470-5526-1_14, © Springer-Verlag Italia 2014

predetermined therapeutic aim to be reached at the lowest human and financial costs, with the fewest undesired effects for the patient and, in particular, with the best compliance and tolerance. There are, however, some general principles that should always be kept in mind:

- the exhaled tidal volume to obtain should always be between 6 and 8 mL/kg in order to obviate difficulty in "emptying" the lungs when exhaling especially in COPD, at the same time as avoiding the application of excessively high insufflation pressures and consequent losses and poor tolerance of NIV;
- the addition of external PEEP in these latter patients can notably reduce the inspiratory effort and improve gas exchange in patients with acute respiratory failure secondary to COPD. Setting an external PEEP (or EPAP) at approximately 70 % of the dynamic PEEPi could reduce the work to which the respiratory pump is subjected by about 40–50 % but, given the difficulty in monitoring PEEPi in clinical practice, great care must be given not to exceed the threshold value represented by the dynamic PEEP, since this would produce the risk of further hyperinflation. The practical advice is never to exceed 6 cmH$_2$O.

The case of the patient with hypoxic respiratory failure is different. In such patients, who have acute pulmonary edema or pneumonia, the level of external PEEP or CPAP should be adjusted according to the SaO$_2$.

14.3   Choose the Ventilator According to the Patient's Need

In the case of severe, hypoxic acute respiratory failure it is preferable to use a ventilator that enables the FiO$_2$ to be set, particularly in the first few hours. Also in the early period and in more instable patients with greater respiratory distress, it is advisable to monitor the patient/ventilator interaction through analysis of the flow and pressure traces and to have the possibility of checking the expired tidal volume. The less restless patient, in whom NIV is used to prevent intubation, often outside a protected environment, can be ventilated with a less sophisticated and manageable ventilator, but one that can in any case compensate for losses.

As said previously, if we want to ventilate a patient with acute pulmonary edema with CPAP, for ease of use we can consider administering the ventilation through a helmet or a simple high flow CPAP system with a traditional interface.

14.4   There is no Single Interface Valid for All Patients

Nature has given us, fortunately or unfortunately, different physical characteristics and for this reason our varied facial features are better adapted to one interface or another. Despite the era of total globalization there are still differences, for example, between the nose of an Asiatic man, that of an Afro-American, or the delicate nose of a female French model. Can we really believe that the same mask will be appropriate for all three cases? This is why it is important to have as broad a range of types and sizes of interfaces as possible, taking into account that all this has a cost for our administrators, but that on the other hand, using NIV avoids other more substantial expenses such as antibiotics to treat cases of intubation-associated pneumonia. It is our duty to make those responsible understand these points. Among the various types of interfaces available on the market, the total face mask and the helmet seem to have features making them suitable for the largest number of patients by, for example, resting directly on the patient's nose.

14.5   Explain What You Want to Do to the Patient

Psychological issues are very important, given that, in contrast to what occurs for intubation, neither neuromuscular blockade nor heavy sedation is used in patients managed with NIV. The patient is therefore an active and not passive part of the ventilatory process during NIV. We like to think that when a patient is intubated, only the clinician's brain is working, whereas when we apply NIV this becomes a means of interaction between the clinician's brain (also through the ventilator) and that of the patient. Obviously, it would be easier for we clinicians to act as "enlightened rulers," but it is our duty to involve our patients in what we are doing.

One of the tricks to facilitate the success of NIV is to explain the technique to patients, especially those without gross changes to the sensorium, before using it. Explaining means simply resting the mask on the patient's face, holding it there with a hand, but not attaching it with elastics or head pieces and in the meantime switching on the ventilator at a low pressure in order to demonstrate what we are going to do. It must be said that sometimes a minimum of psychological warfare can come in hand, for example, recounting the procedure of intubation and its potential side effects if the NIV is not accepted.

14.6   Never Work Alone

The first approach to NIV should never be made by a single person. We shall never tire saying that NIV is not a treatment given by a single person, but the work of a team. The earliest period is the most critical one and the support of at least two people is one of the keys to successful NIV. Ideally, the doctor should first explain the method and then set the ventilator parameters, while the therapist and/or nurse should deal with the choice of the interface, protecting the skin in contact with its surfaces, and applying the interface. Psychological support is an essential part of the work of paramedical staff who are often considered by the patients as emotionally closer to them than is the doctor. The physical presence of a clinician is reassuring for the patient and, at the same time, enables a direct visual assessment of the patient's response.

14.7   Be Aware of Your Limits

A clinician's greatest skill is that of clearly understanding how far he can push without harming the patient. It is not always easy to have good self-awareness and yet this is essential when administering NIV because the greatest risk is that of wasting time futilely by waiting too long before starting intubation. The time factor is crucial in medicine. For example, a study by Esteban and colleagues, in which the effects of NIV in the treatment of post-extubation respiratory failure were evaluated, showed that the ventilated group had a higher mortality rate than the group treated with standard medical therapy for the sole reason that by using NIV the clinicians significantly delayed the use of intubation (Esteban et al. 2004).

There are objective limits to how far a trial of NIV can be pushed; these limits are dictated in part by the patient's disease and in part by more subjective factors. As far as concerns the former, it is worth remembering that the condition of a patient with an exacerbation of COPD usually evolves fairly slowly and that the PaO_2 values rarely fall below dangerous levels because they can be corrected even with a low FiO_2, while a frankly hypoxic patient is at a high risk of deteriorating rapidly. The same applies to the environment in which the NIV is applied. A patient: nurse ratio >1:6–1:8, basic monitoring (i.e., SaO_2) and an old generation ventilator enable a trial of ventilation with the purpose of preventing a worsening of respiratory insufficiency, but certainly not the use of NIV as an alternative to intubation. As far as concerns subjective limitations, we mention lack of familiarity with resuscitation procedures and intubation, a "solo" approach to the patient, tiredness or, even worse, haste, which should all be remembered as limitations. Calling an intensivist when it is still not too late is a sign of respect for him and evidence of your professionalism. Calling him as if to administer the last rites is not only dangerous for you and for him, but is also a demonstration of presumption or lack of responsibility.

14.8   Monitor and Record What You Do

Every therapy worthy of the name must be evaluated through objective parameters. The fortune or misfortune of NIV is that its success or failure is quickly predictable in most cases. The so-called predictors will be discussed later, but what we want to underline here is that with respect to some traditional medical therapies, whose effects can be evaluated sometimes after many minutes (e.g., insulin for glycaemia, corticosteroids or bronchodilators for bronchospasm, diuretics and diuresis), the probable improvements during NIV are seen within a few minutes. For example, a slowing of the respiratory rate and an increase in expired tidal volume are almost inevitably accompanied by a progressive improvement in acidosis and hypercapnia, while a rapid normalization of the SaO_2 as a result of the administration of CPAP in acute pulmonary edema is a sign of a positive response in terms of alveolar recruitment.

We must, however, know which parameter to monitor and "privilege," when to monitor it and above all why to monitor that particular sign. This presumes a minimal knowledge of the physiology of the cardiorespiratory system, which must always form the basis of our choices. Remember to keep track of what has been done and record, write and document the information, perhaps in excel sheets created *ad hoc* according to your needs; this could be useful for you, but above all for the person who will look after your patient when you are no longer there.

Suggested Reading

Ambrosino N, Vagheggini G (2008) Noninvasive positive pressure ventilation in the acute care setting: where are we? Eur Respir J 31(4):874–886

Appendini L, Purro A, Patessio A et al (1996) Partitioning of inspiratory muscle workload and pressure assistance in ventilator-dependent COPD patients. Am J Respir Crit Care Med 154(5):1301–1309

British Thoracic Society Standards of Care Committee (2002) Non-invasive ventilation in acute respiratory failure. Thorax 57(3):192–211

Demoule A, Girou E, Richard JC et al (2006) Benefits and risks of success or failure of noninvasive ventilation. Intensive Care Med 32(11):1756–1765

Elliott MW, Confalonieri M, Nava S (2002) Where to perform noninvasive ventilation? Eur Respir J 19(6):1159–1166

Esteban A, Frutos-Vivar F, Ferguson ND et al (2004) Noninvasive positive-pressure ventilation for respiratory failure after extubation. N Engl J Med 350(24):2452–2460

Esteban A, Ferguson ND, Meade MO et al (2008) Evolution of mechanical ventilation in response to clinical research. Am J Respir Crit Care Med 177(2):170–177

Sinuff T, Cook D, Randall J, Allen C (2000) Noninvasive positive-pressure ventilation: a utilization review of use in a teaching hospital. CMAJ 163(8):969–973

Tricks and Traps of NIV

15

The subtitle of this chapter could be "How details can influence the success of NIV," because sometimes minor changes or precautions can determine whether the attempted ventilation is successful or not.

15.1 Tubing

First of all, we need to clarify the difference between a single limb circuit, a circuit with two limbs and one that has an expiratory valve, as illustrated in Fig. 15.1.

The first ventilators for NIV and most of the home bilevel ones adopt a single circuit, mainly for ease of assembly and of use (the single limb weighs less and is better tolerated by patients who can move in bed). The single limb of these ventilators does not have an expiratory valve and it will, therefore, be your duty to choose a device that prevents the patient from suffocating as a result of re-breathing his own CO_2. Later on in this chapter, there is section on devices to prevent re-breathing.

The ventilators used in intensive care classically have two limbs and for this reason there should not be problems of accumulation of expired gases. One advantage of these disposables is that they enable a more physiological administration of bronchodilating drugs through metered dose inhalers (MDI) or nebulization systems. Furthermore, we should not forget that expired tidal volume can be monitored, and not just estimated, with these systems if there is a pneumotachograph at the Y (where the inspiratory and expiratory limbs meet). The most obvious disadvantages are the weight of the tubing and the fact that they are not very practical.

In theory, a single limb circuit with a true expiratory valve would be the good middle way between the two previously described devices. If fact, this combines the practicality of a single tube with the efficacy of eliminating CO_2 through a real expiratory valve. There are at least two classes of these valves: diaphragm and balloon valves. To the best of our knowledge, only one study, now rather dated

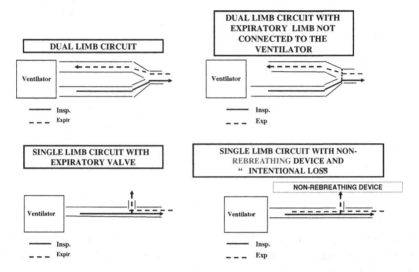

Fig. 15.1 Types of circuits used for NIV

(Lofaso 1998), has compared these different types of valves, finding that there were no significant differences in gas exchange or other parameters between various types of valves. However, there are some models which, because of high expiratory resistances, induce an increase in intrinsic PEEP and, therefore, effort during expiration. As we said earlier, it is not known whether these problems have been resolved in the latest generation ventilators that use this type of valve. Remember that the estimation of tidal volume using a circuit with "non-rebreathing" device is more accurate than that of calculated in a single limb circuit with an expiratory valve.

15.2   The Connections

One of the most annoying things about setting NIV is that when using interfaces or tubes other than those proposed by the manufacturer of the ventilator, it is not always possible to connect the various pieces easily. The suspicion is that we workers in the frontline are being manipulated into using equipment produced by the same company. However, interface X may not be particularly suitable for our patient, who may prefer interface Y which, since it just happens not to be supplied in the kit for that particular ventilator, cannot be connected easily.

Our simple, practical advice is to arrange all the connections that you have on the emergency trolley in order that you do not have to become a do-it-yourself expert when time is money. Avoid situations such as that illustrated in Fig. 15.2 (taken from real life), in which tubes and connections longer than 5–10 cm are put together: this is in order to minimize the dead space and, consequently, the patient's respiratory work load.

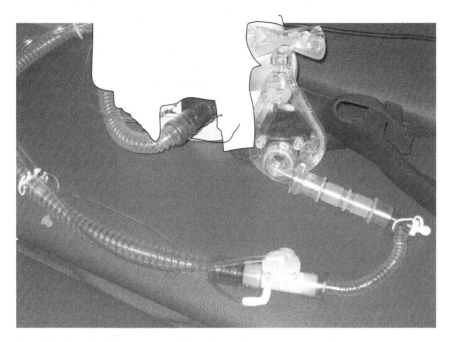

Fig. 15.2 An example of poor assembly of a circuit

A connection 10 cm long with a diameter of 2 cm is already responsible for a considerable increase in dead space. Another simple trick is to have some plasters or tape at hand in order to be able to increase the external diameter of your connection artificially, thereby adapting it to the desired interface, or obtain a connection that is not rigid so that its external diameter can be modified.

15.3 Non-rebreathing Devices

Non-rebreathing devices must only used in true single-limb ventilators, that is, in ventilators that do not have an expiratory valve. Usually, these ventilators are simply called bilevel, and the true inspiratory support is given by the difference between the peak pressure (IPAP) and the expiratory pressure (EPAP). The various companies marketing ventilators have developed several different non-rebreathing devices, the most famous of which are the *whisper swivel®* and the *plateau valve®*.

There is very little research on the efficacy of these devices, except for precisely the two just mentioned. Two studies, which were carried out in the same period by Ferguson and Gilmartin (1995) and Lofaso et al. (1998) showed that when using the whisper swivel, the residual volume of expired air in the circuit at the end of expiration was 55 % of the tidal volume when the ventilator was regulated with a pressure support of 10 cmH$_2$O and a respiratory rate of 15 breaths/minute. It was found that the $PaCO_2$ was about 5 mm Hg lower with the plateau valve than with the whisper swivel; only when the EPAP values were >4 cmH_2O was the problem of rebreathing almost completely eliminated. However, a cross-over study comparing chronic treatment with the two devices did not confirm the difference in efficacy found in the acute situation, suggesting that both devices can be used in long-term ventilation without causing major rebreathing problems.

Unfortunately, as we have already said, these are the only two studies available in the literature, which leads us to make another consideration. When a new drug is introduced onto the market or when the posology of an already used drug is modified, numerous confirmatory studies are necessary and the technical-bureaucratic requirements are rigorous. Ventilators are often life-saving machines and, apart from the CE mark, which is often applied following verification of the electrical characteristics of the machine, nothing else is required by the relevant authorities. We therefore find that we are using new non-rebreathing devices that have almost never been tested *in vivo* with scientific rigor, not to mention the holes made in interfaces that should guarantee removal of CO_2 and that have never been systematically tested on hypercapnic patients. Indeed, one *in vitro* study demonstrated that the so-called 'intentional leaks' in masks could interfere negatively with the function of some ventilators, particularly when the leaks exceed the threshold of 40 L/min. Having said this, we must admit that the equipment we use (ventilators, circuitry, and non-rebreathing devices) is very often clinically effective. The devices, including the masks with holes, introduce losses into the circuit which could interfere with the ventilator's operational algorithm. Within the limits of possible, it is preferable to use a mask and ventilator from the same manufacturer, given that ventilator will very probably have been tested with interfaces produced by the same company. For this reason we advise that you only ever use one device, avoiding the contemporaneous application of a mask with holes together with a non-rebreathing device. If you absolutely have to do this, try to seal the holes in the mask.

15.4 Humidification

The problem of humidification is often underestimated and yet it is very important during both acute and chronic ventilation. Compared to intubation, NIV respects the anatomy and in theory, therefore, the ventilation occurs through the natural pathways. The air that we breathe is, however, normally warmed and humid whereas this is not the case when the air comes from a machine, which produces a flow of cold, dry air. If NIV is applied for only a few hours, as for example in the case of acute pulmonary edema, humidification should not be necessary; however, if the ventilation is protracted for several days, it is very probable that the first side effects will occur. Although these may seem banal, they often determine the tolerance of the NIV. A dry throat, throat pain, a runny nose, nasal congestion, nosebleeds, reactive coughing, hoarseness and in some cases real clots of mucus in the airways, are only some of the irritating complications whose frequency and intensity can be decreased by adding a humidification device to the circuit. There are two main classes of humidifiers for NIV: *heated humidifiers* (HH) and cold humidifiers, also known as *heat and moisture exchangers* (HME).

The former are definitely more complicated to set because they consist of a heating plate on which a bell, filled with water, is placed. The two extremities of the ventilator circuitry are connected to this bell. A thermostat, which can be regulated by the operator, determines the temperature of the water within the bell. The HME, which are commonly called filters, must be divided into two groups: hydroscopic and hydrophobic. The hydrophobic filters have a ceramic fiber membrane that filters bacteria and viruses and allows only partial humidification; these filters are, therefore, only used in the proximal extremity of the ventilator tubes to protect the patient from any contamination. The hydroscopic filter has a polypropylene filter, while its condensation surface is usually made of paper impregnated with $CaCl_2$ and its main role is humidification of the inspired air. It often also filters particles, including bacteria. The most recent HME filters combine the two types of membrane and offer both humidification and filtration, varying, depending on the model, the surface area dedicated to humidification (up to $>2,000$ cm^2) and filtration (up to >500 cm^2). The best filters have a filtration power of >99 % for particles with a diameter between 0.15 and 15 µm. The maximum duration of use proposed for these filters does not usually exceed 24–48 h.

In the light of the foregoing it would seem logical to prefer HME filters because of their ease of use and their relatively limited cost. HME do, however, have notable problems. The first is financial, particularly when considering the chronically ventilated patient; in fact, the filter has to be replaced frequently, while we all know that in most cases the Local Health Authorities provide a few dozen HME a year. The most serious side effect of HME filters is the possible substantial increase in the dead space during NIV, which leads to significant increases in the work of the respiratory system, in the P0.1 and also in the $PaCO_2$ in comparison with humidification systems using HH. These results have been demonstrated by at least two sophisticated physiological studies carried out in France (Jaber et al. 2002; Lellouche et al. 2002).

On the other hand, the potential disadvantages of HH are that these humidifiers are somewhat more complicated to use, there is a possibility of the circuitry becoming contaminated (although, so far, there are no data on a higher incidence of pneumonia in non invasively ventilated patients), and it is sometimes difficult for the patient and the operator to establish a suitable temperature of the circuit. The initial cost is considerably higher than that of the HME, but could be amortized with prolonged use.

If the patient is being ventilated acutely and has a high resistive load with or without hypercapnia, our advice is to use an HH system. In chronic ventilation, a randomized, cross-over study that we performed did not show substantial differences between HME and HH, except for a lower incidence of side effects in the upper airways with the latter system (Nava et al. 2008). To our knowledge there are no studies determining how to obtain better humidification using a helmet.

15.5 Administration of Bronchodilators

Let's clarify one concept immediately: bronchodilators can be given during NIV. The rationale for using these drugs during an episode of acute respiratory failure is based on the fact that they can reduce the work load caused by airway resistance and improve dynamic hyperinflation; their use is, therefore, limited to patients with respiratory distress due to an exacerbation of COPD. In theory, since these patients are not particularly hypoxemic, they could be detached from the ventilator and take beta2-agonists, anticholinergic drugs or steroids through the usual route of administration with an MDI or nebulizer. However, particularly in the early stages of ventilation, the respiratory distress, dyspnea or blunted sensorium could reduce the patient's capacity to take the drugs correctly. For this reason, some studies have focused on the possibility of using bronchodilators during NIV, adapting the settings and method of administration from research carried out in patients ventilated invasively. The first encouraging results were obtained in asthmatic patients using the classical Pressure Support or CPAP and nebulizing the drug in the circuit through an ampoule. Administration of a nebulized drug does, however, create some problems during mechanical ventilation because for an efficacy equivalent to that of a MDI, the risk of contaminating the circuit is higher, the time of administration is longer, and the possibility of interfering with the ventilator's trigger is greater. In clinical practice it is, therefore, preferable to use a MDI, taking into consideration that a large volume spacer has to be introduced into the circuit, as shown in Fig. 15.3, in order to obtain a better distribution of the drug in the bronchi. Our study showed that using a home ventilator with a double circuit, the bronchodilator effect obtained with a salbutamol MDI was comparable to that obtained with nebulization and superior to that produced by a placebo (Nava et al. 2001).

Fig. 15.3 The position of a MDI during NIV

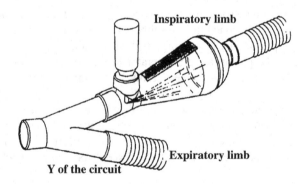

Inspiratory limb

Expiratory limb

Y of the circuit

Study

A later *in vitro* study showed that nebulization is able to produce a reasonable deposition of bronchodilator (>25 %) in the bronchi also when a single limb circuit is used, provided that the ampoule is placed between the non-rebreathing device and the mask, with high inspiratory pressures and low expiratory ones.

15.6   Administration of Oxygen

If your ventilator has a blender and is able to deliver a high flow of oxygen, you will not have any problems. If, however, you use a ventilator without these characteristics, you will have to make do with administering oxygen at a low flow from a gas cylinder, supplied from the wall or a stroller, directly into the ventilator's circuitry.

Thys et al. demonstrated that the FiO_2 delivered depends on various factors, including the position in the circuit at which the oxygen is introduced (Thys et al. 2002). The best position for obtaining a higher FiO_2 is just before the expiratory valve, on the side of the ventilator and not that of the interface. Perhaps more importantly, the FiO_2 is also influenced by the levels of pressure used and, obviously, by the flow of oxygen supplied.

Increasing the inspiratory pressure paradoxically decreases the FiO_2, while relatively high rates of oxygen flow (>6 L/min) are necessary to obtain a FiO_2 >30 %. A practical summary of the results of this study, which can guide our clinical practice, is shown in Fig. 15.4.

		Inspiratory pressure (cmH$_2$O)				
		2	8	12	16	20
	0	19%	20%	21%	21%	21%
	2	26%	24%	24%	24%	22%
O$_2$ flow (L/m)	4	31%	28%	29%	26%	23%
	6	38%	32%	33%	30%	26%
	8	45%	36%	36%	32%	30%
	10	53%	40%	38%	35%	35%
	12	63%	44%	41%	38%	37%
	14	65%	47%	44%	42%	39%

Modified from Thys *et al.* ERJ 2002;19:653-57

Fig. 15.4 Effect of inspiratory pressure on the FiO_2 delivered. Modified from Thys et al. and reproduced with permission of the European Respiratory Society. Eur Respir J April 2002 19:653–657; doi:10.1183/09031936.02.00263102

Suggested Reading

Borel JC, Sabil A, Janssens JP et al (2009) Intentional leaks in industrial masks have a significant impact on efficacy of bilevel noninvasive ventilation: a bench test study. Chest 135(3):669–677

Branconnier MP, Hess D (2005) Albuterol delivery during noninvasive ventilation. Respir Care 50(12):1649–1653

Carlucci A, Schreiber A, Mattei A, Malovini A, Bellinati J, Ceriana P, Gregoretti C (2013) The configuration of bi-level ventilator circuits may affect compensation for non-intentional leaks during volume-targeted ventilation. Intensive Care Med 39(1):59–65

Ceriana P, Navalesi P, Rampulla C et al (2003) Use of bronchodilators during non-invasive mechanical ventilation. Monaldi Arch Chest Dis 59(2):123–127

Chatmongkolchart S, Schettino GP, Dillman C et al (2002) In vitro evaluation of aerosol bronchodilator delivery during non-invasive positive pressure ventilation: effect of ventilator settings and nebulizer position. Crit Care Med 30(11):2515–2519

Craven DE, Goularte TA, Make BJ (1984) Contaminated condensate in mechanical ventilator circuit. A risk factor for nosocomial pneumonia? Am Rev Respir Dis 129(4):625–628

Dhand R, Tobin MJ (1997) Inhaled bronchodilator therapy in mechanically ventilated patients. Am J Respir Crit Care Med 156(1):3–10

Ferguson GT, Gilmartin M (1995) CO2 rebreathing during BiPAP ventilatory asssitance. Am J Respir Crit Care Med 151(4):1126–1135

Hill NS, Carlisle C, Kramer NR (2002) Effect of a nonrebreathing exhalation valve on long-term nasal ventilation using a bilevel device. Chest 122(1):84–91

Jaber S, Chanques G, Matecki S et al (2002) Comparison of the effects of heat and moisture exchangers and heated humidifiers on ventilation and gas exchange during non-invasive ventilation. Intensive Care Med 28(11):1590–1594

Lellouche F, Maggiore SM, Deye N et al (2002) Effect of the humidification device on the work of breathing during noninvasive ventilation. Intensive Care Med 28(11):1582–1589

Lofaso F, Brochard L, Touchard D et al (1995) Evaluation of carbon dioxide rebreathing during pressure support ventilation with airway management system (BiPAP) devices. Chest 108(3):772–778

Lofaso F, Aslanian P, Richard JC et al (1998) Expiratory valves used for home devices: experimental and clinical comparison. Eur Respir J 11(6):1382–1388

Massie CA, Hart RW, Peralez K, Richards GN (1999) Effects of humidification on nasal symptoms and compliance in sleep apnea patients using continuous positive airway pressure. Chest 116(2):403–408

Nava S, Karakurt S, Rampulla C et al (2001) Salbutamol delivery during non-invasive mechanical ventilation in patients with chronic obstructive pulmonary disease: a randomized, controlled study. Intensive Care Med 27(10):1627–1635

Nava S, Cirio S, Fanfulla F (2008) Comparison of two humidification systems for long-term noninvasive mechanical ventilation. Eur Respir J 32(2):460–464

Rakotonanahary D, Pelletier-Fleury N, Gagnadoux F, Fleury B (2001) Predictive factors for the need for additional humidification during nasal continuous positive airways pressure therapy. Chest 119(2):460–465

Schreiber A, Nava S, Ceriana P, Carlucci A (2012) Lack of humidification may harm the patient during continuous positive airway pressure. Br J Anaesth 108(5):884–885

Thys F, Liistro G, Dozin O et al (2002) Determinants of FiO_2 with oxygen supplementation during noninvasive two-level positive pressure ventilation. Eur Respir J 19(4):653–657

Predictors of Failure

Why predictors of failure rather than predictors of success? Because we believe that it is the failure of NIV, above all by culpably and unduly delaying intubation, which determines the outcome of the patient; on the other hand knowing that a patient has a good possibility of success should reassure us but certainly not let us lower our guard.

It should be immediately clarified that the so-called predictors, or perhaps more accurately factors associated with failure, differ greatly between acute hypercapnic respiratory failure due to a pump impairment and hypoxic respiratory failure due to parenchymal problems. As demonstrated by Demoule et al. (2006), a failed attempt at NIV in the former situation is not associated with a higher mortality rate, even if the patient needs intubation, whereas in the case of pure hypoxia, a failed trial of NIV lowers the probability of survival.

16.1 Hypercapnic Respiratory Failure

Table 16.1 lists the possible predictors of failure of NIV during an episode of hypercapnic respiratory failure.

They include clinical parameters, blood-gas values, and mixed indicators. The indices of severity of status on admission to hospital (e.g., SAPS or APACHE) were considered to have a discrete correlation with the outcome of NIV in some studies, whereas no significant correlation was found in others. In any case, it is clear that less severely ill patients (i.e., those with a SAPS II score <30–35 and an APACHE II score <15–20) will have a better outcome. The state of the sensorium is another variable to consider, although taking into account that even comatose patients can be ventilated successfully; the important point is to monitor this index frequently, using the most specific scale possible, such as the Kelly scale.

The possibility of removing bronchial secretions effectively, the tolerance of the NIV, and the presence of massive air losses have been sporadically associated with failure of NIV although it is difficult to determine a threshold level requiring

Table 16.1 Factors associated with failure of NIV

Acute hypercapnic respiratory failure

• Minimal (<0.02) or no change in pH after 1–2 h

• Minimal or no reduction in respiratory rate after 1–2 h

• High severity score at commencement of NIV (i.e. SAPS II>30- APACHE II>20)

• Scarce collaboration or poor tolerance

• Incapacity to remove secretions effectively

Acute hypoxic respiratory failure

• Minimal or no change in the PaO_2/FiO_2 ratio after 1–2 h

• Age >40 years

• High severity score at commencement of NIV (i.e. SAPS II>34)

• Presence of ARDS, CAP and/or sepsis

attention, since most of the studies considered these problems in a dichotomous manner (yes/no).

There is certainly more concordance concerning blood-gas indicators. The pH is the first index to consider, since any changes in the level of $PaCO_2$ are found only later. The absolute value of pH at the time of starting NIV is not necessarily associated with the final outcome since only a few studies have shown a substantial difference between successes and failures.

Certainly, it is intuitive that a patient with a pH <7.25 will be more difficult to ventilate than one with a pH of ~7.30. The single most effective predictor of failure of NIV is definitely change in pH after 1 h of ventilation. A minimal increase (<0.02), no change or, even worse, a decrease in the pH value as the acute response to a trial with NIV is an indicator of almost certain failure.

This does not necessarily mean you have to "wave the white flag" and surrender, but great care must be taken when continuing NIV, perhaps with variations in the parameters, in order not to reach an irreversible clinical condition: the NIV should not be continued for more than another 30–60 min and close monitoring is essential.

The so-called mixed indicators, which take into account several variables, represent an interesting, alternative approach. Certainly the most original and scientifically valid study on this issue is that by Confalonieri et al. (2005), who collected data from more than 1,000 patients and used them to stratify the risk of failure of NIV into three levels corresponding to the colors of a traffic light. The red light, indicating the highest risk of around 70 %, was associated with a pH on admission of <7.25 with an APACHE II score ≥29, a respiratory rate ≥30 breaths per minute, and a score of <11 on the Glasgow Coma Scale. A pH <7.25 after 2 h of ventilation was an indicator of almost certain failure (>90 %). Less severe levels of each of the listed parameters lowered the risk of failure in a manner almost proportional to the number of altered factors and the degree of lesser severity.

It is important to note that while a worsening in the first hours of ventilation is almost always associated with failure of NIV, the opposite—success in those who have dramatic improvement in their clinical conditions after a brief trial—does not hold true. Some years ago, Moretti et al. (2000) showed that a substantial proportion of "early responders" (about 15–20 %) are destined to worsen over time and, therefore, to be intubated or even to die, despite the initial success. The main factors associated with these late failures are comorbidities, in particular hyperglycemia.

So far we have only described and discussed the literature, but these indicators can only provide a rational orientation for our choices, they certainly are not objective guidelines. The success of NIV, just as its failure, depends above all on all those human and organizational variables discussed previously, such as familiarity with the technique, training, environment in which the ventilation takes place, and the number of clinicians involved, factors which cannot easily be quantified and even less so summarized in tables or flow-charts.

16.2 Hypoxic Respiratory Failure

This section of the chapter is much shorter, given the paucity of studies. In fact, there are only four studies focusing on this subject, perhaps because the literature on the use of NIV in hypoxic respiratory failure is much scarcer than that on hypercapnic forms.

In our opinion, the problem of predictors of failure in this field is much more important than in exacerbations of COPD because while the time factor is important in this latter case it is not critical, whereas in the case of the hypoxic patient a delay in instituting alternative forms of ventilation other than NIV can be fatal for the patient. Thus, the speed of decision after a brief trial of NIV is a factor of utmost importance. The decision must be yes or no; "let's see what happens in a while" is not an acceptable choice.

The multicenter study by Antonelli and colleagues in 2001, which involved almost 6,000 patients, showed that age over 40 years, a SAPS II score ≥ 35, the presence of community acquired pneumonia, ARDS and a PaO_2/FiO_2 ratio ≤ 146 after 1 h of NIV were factors independently associated with failure (Antonelli et al. 2001).

Subsequently the same authors focused on patients with ARDS and showed that in this group a SAPS II score ≥ 34 and a PaO_2/FiO_2 ratio ≤ 175 after 1 h were the only independent predictors of failure of NIV (Antonelli et al. 2007). Furthermore, their study showed that patients who were intubated were, on average, older and required higher levels of external PEEP and/or Pressure Support.

In a relatively small, consecutive series of hypoxic patients, Rana et al. (2006) demonstrated that the presence of shock, metabolic acidosis, and a low PaO_2/FiO_2 ratio were factors predicting failure of NIV. Demoule et al. (2006), analyzing data from 70 French intensive care units, concluded that the failure of NIV in hypoxic patients was correlated with a high mortality (OR of 3.24), once again confirming that one must be very prudent when treating such patients with NIV.

In conclusion, there are easily measurable clinical factors that can rapidly alert a clinician to the possible failure of NIV and lead him to a quick decision to intubate the patient. However, we do note that the umbrella term of hypoxia covers numerous pathologies with very different pathogenic mechanisms and their responses to NIV could, therefore, be markedly different. For example, as already said earlier, a given PaO_2/FiO_2 ratio in a patient with acute pulmonary edema has a completely different meaning from the same ratio in a patient with ARDS.

Suggested Reading

Ambrosino N, Foglio K, Rubini F et al (1995) Non-invasive mechanical ventilation in acute respiratory failure due to chronic obstructive pulmonary disease: correlates for success. Thorax 50(7):755–757

Antonelli M, Conti G, Moro ML (2001) Predictors of failure of noninvasive positive pressure ventilation in patients with acute hypoxemic respiratory failure: a multi-center study. Intensive Care Med 27(11):1718–1728

Antonelli M, Conti G, Esquinas A et al (2007) A multiple-center survey on the use in clinical practice of noninvasive ventilation as a first-line intervention for acute respiratory distress syndrome. Crit Care Med 35(1):18–25

Carlucci A, Richard JC (2001) Noninvasive versus conventional mechanical ventilation. An epidemiological survey. Am J Respir Crit Care Med 163(4):874–880

Carlucci A, Delmastro M, Rubini F et al (2003) Changes in the practice of non-invasive ventilation in treating COPD patients over 8 years. Intensive Care Med 29(3):419–425

Confalonieri M, Garuti G, Cattaruzza MS et al (2005) Italian noninvasive positive pressure ventilation (NPPV) study group. A chart of failure risk for noninvasive ventilation in patients with COPD exacerbation. Eur Respir J 25:348–355

Demoule A, Girou E, Richard JC et al (2006) Benefits and risks of success or failure of noninvasive ventilation. Intensive Care Med 32(11):1756–1765

Meduri GU, Abou-Shala N, Fox RC et al (1991) Noninvasive face mask mechanical ventilation in patients with acute hypercapnic respiratory failure. Chest 100(2):445–454

Moretti M, Cilione C, Tampieri A et al (2000) Incidence and causes of non-invasive mechanical ventilation failure after initial success. Thorax 55(10):819–825

Nava S, Carlucci A (2002) Non-invasive pressure support ventilation in acute hypoxemic respiratory failure: common strategy for different pathologies? Intensive Care Med 28(9):1205–1207

Nava S, Ceriana P (2004) Causes of failure of noninvasive mechanical ventilation. Respir Care 49(3):295–303

Rana S, Jenad H, Gay PC et al (2006) Failure of non-invasive ventilation in patients with acute lung injury: observational cohort study. Crit Care 10(3):R79

Soo Hoo GW, Santiago S, Williams AJ (1994) Nasal mechanical ventilation for hypercapnic respiratory failure in chronic obstructive pulmonary disease: determinants of success and failure. Crit Care Med 22(8):1253–1261

Where to Ventilate a Patient with NIV

17

The answer to this question is not easy. Someone interested in being politically correct (and we are not) would say "anywhere that there is someone who knows how to do it." We must rectify this misconception immediately. The ideal place to apply NIV depends almost entirely on the timing of its use. Figure 17.1 is an attempted diagram of the indications for NIV and places in which to apply it.

Our diagram does not, of course, take into account the true local conditions, the real doctor/patient ratio and, more importantly, the nurse/patient ratio, the monitoring system available, and the experience acquired by the team over time.

There are diseases for which patients are now almost never admitted to an intensive care unit, such as pulmonary edema and mild exacerbations of COPD, because these usually respond so well that they can be treated outside protected environments; the former case can even be treated directly in the patient's home or in an ambulance.

Then there are particular conditions, such as the immunocompromised patient, in which it is better to avoid admission to an environment at high risk of infections, or terminal care, in which the NIV has only a palliative purpose and the patient and his relatives need privacy that is unlikely to be possible in an intensive care setting.

Besides experience with NIV, what makes the great difference between the various settings in which NIV is used is the monitoring system and the number of staff. In France, respiratory intensive care units or subintensive care units are classified into levels depending on the system of monitoring available; a similar strategy is also being attempted in Italy in accordance with the guidelines from the Italian Association of Hospital Pneumologists (AIPO); a patient may only be ventilated non invasively if a minimum set of instruments is available. In an English study of a few years ago, it was calculated that the annual prevalence of patients requiring NIV in a typical hospital in the United Kingdom is 75/100,000 among men and 57/100,000 among women. According to the authors, this means that each district general hospital should have a service dedicated specifically to NIV.

Openness to the world of NIV does not necessarily mean that the doctor must know how to intubate, as if this was the only limit to consider, but rather that he is

S. Nava and F. Fanfulla, *Non Invasive Artificial Ventilation*,
DOI: 10.1007/978-88-470-5526-1_17, © Springer-Verlag Italia 2014

able to manage the preceding stages skillfully (the famous barrier of how far to persist with NIV) and any stages after intubation (application of invasive ventilation and any treatment of its consequences). In the case that the ideal structure does not exist, which is the situation in the majority of cases, it is to be hoped that the doctor, whatever his qualification (pneumologist, internist), can obtain help in real time from a colleague specialized in reanimation. For this reason, it is at least theoretically logical that NIV is administered in an area close to an intensive care unit.

In most cases the ideal place in which a patient should be treated is a respiratory intensive care unit, a subintensive care unit or a 'step-down' unit, however you wish to call it. Documents from AIPO and the European Respiratory Society (ERS) define three standards of respiratory intensive care unit based primarily on the monitoring, the type of ventilation possible besides NIV, the qualifications of the staff, the possibility of carrying out invasive procedures and perhaps physiotherapy. This has already been discussed and will be examined again in the chapter on monitoring, but we want to list here the structural features of a respiratory intensive care unit.

First of all, the structure and location of these units must take into account the pre-established purposes, which are ventilation therapy, non invasive monitoring, and free access to physiotherapists and relatives. A respiratory intensive care unit must be architectonically different from a traditional pneumology ward in that the access should be controlled and independent and have a minimum total area about three times greater than that of the body surface area of each, individual patient.

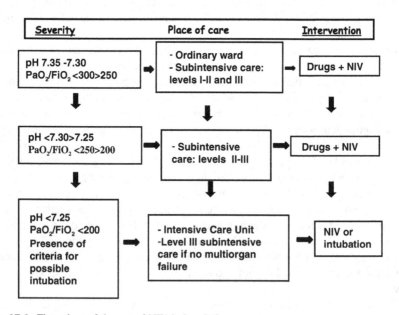

Fig. 17.1 Flow-chart of the use of NIV in hospital

The distinction from a traditional intensive care unit lies in the fact that the intensive respiratory care unit has a so-called open arrangement, which, while essentially retaining the same aseptic characteristics, enables controlled entry of the relatives directly involved in the rehabilitation programs. The main disadvantages of this type of structure are the lack of privacy and a potential increased risk of cross-infections, although this latter has not been demonstrated to be the case.

The ideal number of beds for this structure was stated by the AIPO in their guidelines on respiratory intensive care units to be 4–6 beds for a hospital with a capacity for more than 500 patients and 8 beds for a hospital with a capacity for more than 1,000 patients, or 1–2 beds for every 100,000 inhabitants. In the ideal structure, the area per patient should be 28 m^2 for a single room and 25 m^2 for shared rooms, including the space required for paramedical purposes and relatives' needs. In the case of a shared room, the bathroom must be spacious and have a so-called ante-room with sanitary installations including a bath for the handicapped. The access to the respiratory intensive care unit must allow easy passage of a bed and all the mobile equipment and instruments necessary, such as a portable X-ray machine, dialysis, and an echocardiograph.

The single or isolation rooms, usually reserved for immunocompromised patients, should have an ante-room of about 2.5 m^2 to allow visitors to wash their hands and put on a gown.

The structure behind and to either side of each bed should provide electricity sockets, compressed air, oxygen, a vacuum (for aspiration), and shelves where the ventilators and monitoring equipment can be placed; these should be articulated and suspended to enable rational positioning depending on the space needed for the medical and paramedical procedures. It is useful to provide space for at least two people behind the bed in order to enable help in the case of intubation, introduction of a central venous catheter, or resuscitation procedures. The bed should be mobile, with adjustable angulation controlled electronically and it should be possible to remove the bedhead.

A generator should be able to supply electricity automatically if a loss of current lasts for more than 5s. As far as concerns the gases and heating system, it is worth standardizing some parameters, such as:

- vacuum: negative pressure of 500 mmHg, with a constant flow of 40 L/m;
- oxygen: pressure of 5 bar, which should remain constant when the flow is 20 L/m at each output with all the outputs in use;
- compressed air: pressure of 5 bar, which should remain constant when the flow is 20 L/m at each output with all the outputs in use;
- ventilation: air filtered at 99 % for particles of a diameter of 5 mm; air-conditioning system with a relative humidity of 30–50 %;
- heating: 18–27 °C.

Each respiratory intensive care unit should include an operational center for nurses, with individual monitoring, and be equipped with a telephone, storage of disposable supplies for first aid, a defibrillator, and a small pharmacy.

Table 17.1 Factors to consider when deciding "where to ventilate"

- Severity of the patient's condition

- Type of monitoring

- Patient/nurse ratio

- "Weaning test" (i.e., in how much time a patient's clinical state and blood gases deteriorate once the interface has been removed)

- The patient's capacity and possibility to ask for help in the case of an emergency

- The clinical staff's experience and skill in administering NIV

- Types of ventilator and oxygen sources available (i.e., high vs. low flow O_2)

- Numbers, sizes, and types of interfaces available

- Proximity to the intensive care unit

The storage space for the supplies must be easily reached by the medical and paramedical staff and there must be a "satellite" pharmacy, a refrigerator for storing blood samples, and equipment for emergencies.

In brief, when we are going to ventilate a patient non invasively, we must always ask ourselves a few simple questions and answer honestly, considering our limitations and our skills. Table 17.1 could be some help in this sense.

Suggested Reading

Byrick RJ, Power JD, Ycas JO, Brown KA (1986) Impact of an intermediate care area on ICU utilization after cardiac surgery. Crit Care Med 14(10):869–872

Bone RC, Balk RA (1988) Noninvasive respiratory care unit: a cost effective solution for the future. Chest 93(2):390–394

Confalonieri M, Gorini M, Ambrosino N et al (2001) Respiratory intensive care unit in Italy: a national census and prospective cohort study. Thorax 56(5):373–378

Corrado A, Roussos C, Ambrosino N et al (2002) Respiratory intermediate care units: a European survey. Eur Respir J 20(5):1343–1350

French Multicentric Group of ICU research (1989) Description of various types of intensive and intermediate care units in France. Intensive Care Med 15(4):260–265

Fracchia C, Ambrosino N (1994) Location and architectural structure of IICU. Monaldi Arch Chest Dis 49(6):496–498

Iapichino G, Apolone G, Melotti R et al (1994) Intermediate intensive units: definition, legislation and need in Italy. Monaldi Arch Chest Dis 49(6):493–495

Iapichino G, Radrizzani D, Ferla L et al (2002) Description of trends in the course of illness of critically ill patients: markers of intensive care organization and performance. Intensive Care Med 28(7):985–989

Laufman H (1986) Planning and building the ICU: problems of design, infection control and cost/benefit. In: Reis Miranda DL (ed) The ICU: a cost/benefit analysis. Congress Series. Excerpta Medica, Amsterdam

Nasraway SA, Cohen IL, Dennis RC et al (1998) Guidelines on admission and discharge for adult intermediate care units: American College of Critical Care Medicine of the Society of Critical Care Medicine. Crit Care Med 26(3):607–610

Nava S, Confalonieri M, Rampulla C (1998) Intermediate respiratory intensive care units in Europe: a European perspective. Thorax 53(9):798–802

Plant PK, Owen JL, Elliott MW (2000) One year period prevalence study of respiratory acidosis in acute exacerbations of COPD: implications for the provision of non-invasive ventilation and oxygen administration. Thorax 55(7):550–554

Valentini I, Pacilli AMS, Carbonara P et al (2013) Influence of the admission pattern on the outcome of patients admitted to a RICU: does the step-down admission differ from a step-up one? Resp. Care 58(12):210–220

Monitoring During NIV

18

The minimum monitoring is that appropriate for the severity of the patient's condition, taking into account that clinical conditions can change rapidly. It does not, therefore, make sense to have invasive hemodynamic monitoring available when we are treating a simple, early stage of an exacerbation of COPD, just as it would be unthinkable to use NIV in a patient with pneumonia and severe hypoxia with only pulse oximetry available. It would obviously be desirable to work in a structure that has an integrated system of non invasive and invasive monitoring in order not to have to transfer the patient to another structure if his condition worsens. Outside intensive care units, this is possible only in third level respiratory intensive care units.

The main feature distinguishing a respiratory intensive care unit from normal intensive care units is that non invasive techniques of ventilation and monitoring patients with respiratory failure are privileged in the former; this approach does not, however, exclude recourse to invasive methods of ventilation and/or monitoring if the situation necessitates it. The concept of non invasive ventilation and monitoring enables ventilation therapy to be instituted in structures that are not highly specialized such as classical respiratory wards and the casualty department, as well as in wards for specific disorders, such as cardiology, neurology, oncology, and palliative care wards.

According to published data, a reduction in invasive maneuvers reduces the risk of infections and trauma (e.g., pneumothorax), shortens the time spent in hospital, improves the compliance of patients, and lowers the overall costs of patients' care.

The critical situation of a ventilated patient obliges careful monitoring which enables us to obtain:

- acceptable standards of diagnosis, treatment, and management;
- better understanding of the pathophysiology of the acutely ill patient;
- an evaluation of the therapeutic response and prognosis;
- prompt detection of any changes (for better or worse) of the patient's clinical and pathophysiological conditions.

S. Nava and F. Fanfulla, *Non Invasive Artificial Ventilation*,
DOI: 10.1007/978-88-470-5526-1_18, © Springer-Verlag Italia 2014

We can schematically distinguish the parameters used to monitor a patient during NIV according to the levels of intensity of care and monitoring proposed by the various scientific societies into:

1. level I, routinely used, essential parameters characterized by:
   • ease of use;
• relatively low cost;
• "nonspecialist" interpretation;
• minimal invasiveness;
2. level II, partially invasive or non invasive, parameters generally characterized by:
   • higher cost;
• less continuous use;
• more specialist interpretation;
• possible relative invasiveness for the patient;
3. level III, invasive, characterized by:
   • high cost;
• need for specialized, expert staff (true ICU setting).

In accordance with the AIPO guidelines, level I monitoring is carried out for all non invasively ventilated patients. This does not, however, exclude an almost routine use of methods for level II and III monitoring.

18.1   Level I Monitoring

18.1.1 Physical Examination

A clinical examination of the patient may reveal physical signs of the disease and feed-back on the response to treatment. The physical examination in critically ill patients is aimed principally at detecting premonitory or actual signs of acute respiratory distress and controlling the vital signs, which provide a clinical picture of the patient's state of health. Signs of respiratory muscle distress that must be carefully looked for are:
• paradoxical abdominal movements;
• thoracic-abdominal alternation;
• activation of the accessory inspiratory muscles;
• tone of the abdominal muscles during the respiratory cycle;
• Hoover's sign (paradoxical inward movement of the last ribs during inspiration);
• tachypnea. Other fundamental parameters of the physical examination are:
• body temperature, measured at least four times in 24 h;
• respiratory rate (see later);
• 24-h urine output or hourly urine output by bladder catheterization

- state of consciousness (sensorium) of the patient, which can be evaluated by various scales of severity, such as the Glasgow Coma Scale (GCS), whose score is incorporated in the APACHE II evaluation, and the Kelly scale.

18.1.2 Respiratory Rate

Expressed in breaths per minute, this often undervalued parameter correlates well with the degree of respiratory distress, but is unfortunately almost never recorded on the patient's temperature chart. A high respiratory rate (>30 breaths/minute) which does not alter following sensorial or emotional stimuli is an indirect sign that, from a respiratory point of view, the patient is working at the upper limits of his potential.

18.1.3 Dyspnea

It is almost scandalous how we pneumologists often undervalue this parameter which gives us a measure of the respiratory distress or, as we like to call it, of the "pain of the respiratory system." In oncology and palliative care pain is measured as frequently as several times a day to guide drug dosing and any therapeutic choices, using the same scales that we use. These are the Borg scale or visual analogue scale (VAS), shown in Fig. 18.1. These scales are very easy to use, provided the patient does not have profound sensorial alterations.

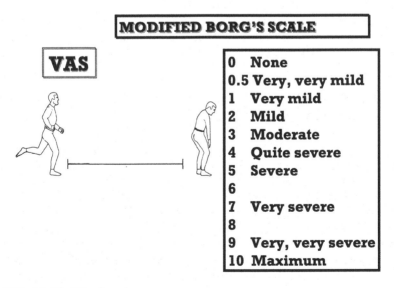

Fig. 18.1 Modified Borg's scale

18.1.4 Blood-Gas Analyses and Related Parameters

Analysis of the blood gases supplies essential data on the overall efficiency of respiration. It is the main examination to evaluate the efficacy of mechanical ventilation because of its ease of use and the reliability of the information it gives on:
- alveolar ventilation, from measuring the $PaCO_2$;
- gas exchange in relation to the FiO_2, from measuring the PaO_2;
- acid–base balance, from also measuring the pH and, indirectly, bicarbonates and the base excess.

The arterial blood gases should be analyzed at predetermined intervals in the first few hours of NIV and then at least once a day and, possibly, after every change in FiO_2 and modality of ventilation.

18.1.5 Pulse Oximetry

This technique for measuring percentage SaO_2 exploits the different spectra of absorption or reflection of light (red light at 660 nm; infrared at 900 nm) by oxygenated hemoglobin and deoxygenated (reduced) hemoglobin. The SaO_2 should be considered a vital parameter and monitored continuously in the first 24 h in patients in respiratory intensive care units because, by supplying a continuous measurement which can be recorded and used to trigger alarms, it can overcome the limits inherent in the intermittent nature of blood-gas analyses. The equipment is very simple, relatively cheap, and no particular training is necessary in order to use it. The limitations of pulse oximetry measurements are that:
- precise readings for PaO_2 values between 80 and 160 mmHg are impossible;
- SaO_2 values <60 % are underestimated;
- the measurement is influenced by the patient's movements, degree of tissue perfusion, presence of jaundice or skin pigmentation, levels of methemoglobin, levels of carboxyhemoglobin, and diffusion of light from environmental sources.

18.1.6 Basic Monitoring of Cardiovascular Function (ECG and Non Invasively Measured Systemic Arterial Blood Pressure)

Disorders of heart rhythm are frequently found in the later stages of advanced chronic respiratory disorders or at any case in situations of chronic hypoxia. The possibility of identifying such arrhythmias visually should be an integrated part of monitoring systems in whatever way they are configured and for this reason continuous monitoring is indicated for at least the first 24 h. A full ECG trace should be printed at least every 24 h.

There is equipment for monitoring systemic blood pressure which uses normal sphygmomanometer blood pressure cuffs that are inflated regularly and record the blood pressure automatically. There are also instruments based on the plethysmographic method which enable continual (pulsed), non invasive determination of the blood pressure; however, these instruments only give a qualitative assessment, since the measurements are affected by movements of the finger which has been cuffed, and cannot, therefore, be considered reliable for use in intensive care.

18.1.7 Exhaled Tidal Volume

In patients undergoing mechanical ventilation, respiratory function can be analyzed easily with simply and widely available equipment: a pneumotachograph to measure the flow (V), a flow signal integrator to obtain the volume (TV) or a simple portable spirometer (Wright type).

In the vast majority of cases, continuous or periodic measurements of dynamic lung volumes are possible and are simple, basic parameters of diagnostic and clinical utility. In particular, expired tidal volume is a very important parameter to measure during NIV because it reflects the patient's alveolar ventilation better than the inspired volume set on the ventilator (in the case of A/C volume ventilation), which is susceptible to losses due to poor positioning of the mask. Many of the common ventilators for NIV allow real-time monitoring of the expired tidal volume and even the losses. Some of the single limb ventilators can also record these parameters, albeit from an algorithm that estimates them, not from direct measurements. The reliability of these measures varies greatly from ventilator to ventilator. This is a critical problem because, beyond controlling the electrical component of the equipment, the regulatory bodies charged with controlling ventilators very rarely ensure that the values reported by the monitoring system are accurate. Perhaps the most emblematic case is that reported by Lofaso et al., who showed that, also *in vitro*, the setting of a tidal volume established in controlled mode varied greatly depending on the level of resistance (which should not occur because in volume ventilation the tidal volume is an independent variable!) and on the ventilator used (Lofaso et al. 2000).

18.1.8 Prognostic Scores

The Acute Physiological Score and Chronic Health Evaluation (APACHE) score and the Simplified Acute Physiological Score (SAPS), both of which have been revised and updated over the years, take into account numerous physiological variables, the age of the patient and his preceding general state of health. The values of the APACHE and SAPS correlate fairly well with patients' survival data. In any case, they give an instantaneous and fairly complete 'photograph' of the patient's general condition.

We should always remember that acute respiratory failure is not the only problem to consider in many of the patients who come to our attention with numerous comorbid conditions, especially if they have a chronic respiratory disorder.

Table 18.1 Scale of delirium according to the Intensive Care Delirium Screening checklist

(1) *Altered level of consciousness*
(a) coma = no further evaluation
(b) somnolence or over-alertness = 1 point
(2) *Inattention*: in the presence of (a) difficulty in following a conversation; (b) easily distracted, (c) difficulty in shifting focuses = 1 point
(3) *Disorientation*: any obvious mistake in time, place or person = 1 point
(4) *Hallucinations* = 1 point
(5) *Psychomotor agitation or retardation* = 1 point
(6) *Inappropriate speech or mood* = 1 point
(7) *Major sleep/wake cycle disturbance* = 1 point
(8) Symptom fluctuation = 1 point

Delirium is diagnosed in the presence of a score ≥4. A score of 2 or 3 signifies a borderline case

18.1.9 Delirium

There have been numerous studies on delirium in patients admitted to an intensive care unit or who are being ventilated mechanically. Frank delirium is associated with prolonged mechanical ventilation and protracted admissions to hospital. Furthermore, interfering with a patient's intellectual capacities can be a major limitation to the use of NIV. It is, therefore, important to recognize the symptoms of the syndrome early, which can be done using simple scales which, like the Intensive Care Delirium Screening Checklist (ICDSC) presented in Table 18.1, can be filled in easily by nursing staff.

18.2 Level II Monitoring

18.2.1 Measure of the Efficacy of the Respiratory Muscles

The maximum inspiratory pressure (MIP) is the negative pressure that develops at the mouth during an inspiratory effort performed with the airways closed and maintained for at least 1 s (it is, therefore, useful to monitor the trace constantly). This measurement is performed preferably at the functional residual capacity if it possible to determine, by spirometry, the tidal volume or, if not, at the residual volume. It may be difficult in the first few hours of positive pressure NIV in the acutely ill patient and for as long as the patient is suffering major respiratory distress. When possible, the MIP should be measured every 24 h.

The same comments concerning MIP also apply to the maximal expiratory pressure (MEP), remembering that in the absence of spirometric information, the procedure should be performed at total lung capacity.

While the MIP gives us an indication of the potential residual capacity of the respiratory muscles as generators of force (although in the absence of an equally important parameter: the proportion of this maximal force that is used in each spontaneous breath), the MEP gives us information on the function of the expiratory muscles that are recruited when, for example, the patient wants to remove secretions. For this purpose, measuring the peak expiratory flow may be an easier alternative to MEP.

18.2.2 Transcutaneous Monitoring of Gases (PtcCO$_2$ and PtcO$_2$)

Continuous transcutaneous measurement of PCO$_2$ and PO$_2$ is useful after the very earliest stage of acute respiratory failure to control the efficacy of the ventilator at improving gas exchange during sleep.

The most recent electrodes for transcutaneous monitoring of blood gases incorporate, in a single miniaturized system, the Clark's polarographic system for measuring PtcCO$_2$ and the Stowe-Severinghaus electrode modified for the measurement of PtcO$_2$. The operative principle is based on the creation of an area of cutaneous hyperemia that promotes vasodilatation of the capillaries. The value of the PtcCO$_2$ is usually overestimated but the error remains constant throughout the recording; in contrast the PtcO$_2$ in the adult is underestimated by about 20 % with respect to real PaO$_2$ values. However, the electrode must be moved after a few hours and the instrument must be re-calibrated every time the position of the electrode is changed. The most important factors that reduce the accuracy of transcutaneous measurements of gases are the thickness of the skin, the presence of abundant subcutaneous adipose tissue and the state of the blood circulation below the electrode.

18.2.3 Capnometry and Capnography

Non invasive measurements of the concentration of CO$_2$ in exhaled air enables the PaCO$_2$ and, therefore, the PaCO$_2$ to be monitored over time. Capnometry can be used to visualize the concentration of CO$_2$ in the expired air breath by breath, while capnography also provides a trace of the wave of expired CO$_2$ with indirect information on the patient's ventilatory status. These instruments exploit various different forms of technology, from the most sophisticated and expensive mass spectrometry to the more widespread and less expensive ultrared absorption spectrophotometry. The measurements can be performed in main-stream or side-stream modality, detecting the end-tidal CO$_2$ (ETCO$_2$) via nasal catheters. The correlation between the concentration of CO$_2$ at peak expiration, i.e., the ETCO$_2$, and the PaCO$_2$ is usually not particularly good, particularly in patients with obstructive disease and in those with an increased dead space.

In normal subjects the PaCO$_2$ is from 1 to 5 mmHg higher than the ETCO$_2$.

18.2.4 The Alveolar-Capillary O$_2$ Gradient

This is a measure of the efficiency of gas exchange and in particular the capacity of alveolar-capillary diffusion of oxygen, determined non invasively from the formula for alveolar gases $(A - a)O_2 = FiO_2(Patm - PH_2O) - PaCO_2/0.8$. Many commercially available blood-gas analyzers supply the values.

18.2.5 Peripheral Venous Pressure

This is measured by drum-type catheters placed in a peripheral vein. However, for a more correct interpretation of venous pressures, it is better to use the levels in a central vein, which means running the typical risks of an invasive procedure.

18.2.6 Invasive Arterial Blood Pressure

This is measured after having cannulated a peripheral artery and allows us to monitor systemic arterial blood pressure in real time. Cannulation is also useful in the case that the patient requires frequent blood-gas analyses.

18.2.7 Static Lung Volumes

Static lung volumes are measured once the patient is able to breathe autonomously and is in a stable clinical condition. It is particularly important to determine the degree of static hyperinflation by measuring the residual functional capacity and the residual volume.

18.2.8 Color-Doppler Echocardiography

Echocardiography is a reliable, non invasive method of monitoring, in particular for a qualitative evaluation of right and left ventricular volumes and of left ventricular ejection fraction; its quantitative accuracy is under debate. In fact, compared to ventriculography, echocardiography tends to underestimate the left end-diastolic ventricular volume; this underestimation can lead to imprecision in the calculation of the stroke volume. Echocardiography provides other morphofunctional information (duration of the pre-ejection period and the relaxation time of the right ventricle, septal thickness, and dimensions of the right atrium) and indirectly enables the pulmonary vascular resistance to be calculated: a good correlation has been demonstrated between pulsed Doppler measurements of peak acceleration time (TaccP) or tricuspid regurgitation and pulmonary artery pressure measured by cardiac catheterization. Echocardiography may be difficult to perform in patients being ventilated mechanically because of the poor technical quality of the images. In these cases, the examination may be carried out with a trans-esophageal method which, although it provides better quality images, does involve some risks related to the invasiveness of the technique.

18.2.9 Ultrasonography

This imaging technique is currently very fashionable in the fields of resuscitation and pneumology. It is particularly useful for the diagnosis of pleural effusions and their treatment (i.e., needle guidance) and for the diagnosis of a pneumothorax. Furthermore, it has become the gold standard method for guiding the placement of central venous catheters. It seems destined to become an indispensable technique in pneumology in the coming years.

18.3 Level III Invasive or Highly Specialized Monitoring

18.3.1 Measurements of Respiratory Mechanics

Some dynamic parameters of respiratory mechanics can be monitored in patients being ventilated non invasively using portable instruments designed specifically for this purpose. These instruments incorporate a pneumotachograph, gastro-esophageal probes, and an airway pressure detector. These partially invasive methods can provide a real-time, and therefore dynamic, record of pulmonary resistances, chest cage resistance, compliance, dynamic intrinsic PEEP (PEEPi, dyn), and the respiratory work performed by the patient. In patients with acute respiratory distress syndrome, setting the ventilator by measuring esophageal pressure was found to be extremely effective in improving oxygenation and compliance compared to the results obtained with normal practice. Almost all these parameters are derived from the recording of the transdiaphragmatic pressure (Pdi), which is recorded by a balloon-catheter system connected to a pressure transducer. Two catheters are placed, one in the distal third of the esophagus (to measure the esophageal pressure, Pes) and the other in the stomach (to measure gastric pressure, Pga). The Pdi is obtained from the following formula: $Pdi = Pga - (-Pes)$.

The Pdi gives us information that is useful for setting the extrinsic PEEP, since the intrinsic PEEP can be measured on this signal, and for Pressure Support, since it supplies the reduction in inspiratory effort under ventilation in real time. Furthermore, the maximum Pdi can be measured with two distinct procedures, the so-called combined maneuver (maximum inspiratory effort of the thoracic component and expulsive force of the abdominal component) and the 'sniff,' obtained by a vigorous inspiration through the nose. The former maneuver mainly reflects the strength of the diaphragm, while the latter reflects the strength of the diaphragm and all the other inspiratory muscles.

18.3.2 Electromyography of the Respiratory Muscles

This is used to measure neuromuscular activity and is recorded through surface electrodes or via an esophageal catheter. Electromyography of the diaphragm (Edi) can be used to determine the presence or absence of electrical activity (in the case of suspected paralysis), or to determine, in a non invasive manner, the reduction in amplitude of the signal following the use of ventilation.

18.3.3 Inductive Plethysmography

This is used to obtain an indirect measure of lung volumes and respiratory pattern through the determination of thoraco-abdominal movements. It is performed with two bands placed around the chest cage and the abdomen. It is difficult to calibrate (isovolumetric maneuver), but can be used to evaluate respiratory timing (Ti, Te, Ttot, RR), for a qualitative analysis of the breathing (paradoxical movements, thoraco-abdominal alternation) or to calculate rough changes in ventilation (for example, between spontaneous breathing and ventilation therapy, during the passage from assisted to spontaneous ventilation). It is not very reliable at quantifying the tidal volume in milliliters because of numerous variables that must be taken into consideration, and the absolute values of the end-expiratory lung volume should, therefore, be interpreted with care.

18.3.4 Hemodynamics

Pulmonary artery catheterization is an expensive, invasive technique, and specific skills are necessary both to perform it and interpret its results. It can only be carried out in a ICU or respiratory intensive care setting. Direct measurement of right-sided pressures is indicated in the case of acute decompensation of chronic cor pulmonale and in severe pulmonary hypertension in order to evaluate the efficacy of the therapy. It is also useful for making a differential diagnosis between cor pulmonale and biventricular or left heart failure. Furthermore, it enables samples to be taken for the determination of central venous oxygen saturation (SvO$_2$). Besides the classical Swan-Ganz catheter, there is a microcatheter that can be introduced peripherally, without requiring radioscopic control; this device is named after its inventor, Grandjean, and appears to be particularly useful in patients in whom invasive procedures must be limited such as conscious patients being ventilated non invasively.

18.3.5 Mixed Venous Blood O$_2$ Saturation and Venous Admixture

A useful indicator of an abnormal ventilation/perfusion ratio is the measurement of the physiological shunt (also called 'venous admixture'), for which a sample of mixed venous blood is necessary. This sample must be taken from the distal lumen of the Swanz–Ganz catheter, with the balloon deflated, checking on the screen that the pressure curve is that of the pulmonary artery and aspirating gently to avoid collecting capillary blood. The same method can be used to calculate the O$_2$ saturation in mixed venous blood (SvO$_2$). The SvO$_2$ correlates better with PvO$_2$ than the SaO$_2$ does with the PaO$_2$, since its values fall in the rising part of the SatHbO$_2$ curve. In this part of the curve, the relationship between the SvO$_2$ and the mixed venous oxygen tension (PvO$_2$) is linear and, therefore, a change in 1 mmHg of PvO$_2$ is associated with a change of about 2 % in the SvO$_2$. There are now catheters that enable continuous monitoring of the SvO$_2$ by a spectrophotometric method. The pathological conditions associated with a decrease in SvO$_2$ are drops in cardiac output, SaO$_2$, and hemoglobin concentration and an increase in oxygen consumption. An increase in the SvO$_2$ is usually accompanied by an increase in oxygen delivery, a decrease in oxygen consumption and its extraction by tissues, a left-to-right shunt within the heart and severe mitral regurgitation.

Suggested Reading

Aubier M, Murciano D, Lecocquic Y et al (1985) Bilateral phrenic stimulation: a simple technique to assess diaphragmatic fatigue in humans. J Appl Physiol 58(1):58–64

Bellemare F, Grassino A (1983) Force reserve of the diaphragm in patients with chronic obstructive pulmonary disease. J Appl Physiol 55(1 Pt 1):8–15

Bergeron N, Dubois MJ, Dumont M et al (2001) Intensive care delirium screening checklist: evaluation of a new screening tool. Intensive Care Med 27(5):859–864

Bone RG (1990) Monitoring respiratory and hemodynamic function in the patient with respiratory failure. In: Kirby RR, Banner MJ, Downs JB (eds) Clinical applications of ventilatory support. Churchill Livingstone Med, New York

Carlucci A, Schreiber A, Mattei A et al (2013) The configuration of bi-level ventilator circuits may affect compensation for non-intentional leaks during volume-targeted ventilation Intensive Care Med 39(1):59–65

Ceriana P, Fanfulla F, Mazzacane F et al (2010) Delirium in patients admitted to a step-down unit: analysis of incidence and risk factors. J Crit Care 25(1):136–143

Corrado A, Ambrosino N, Rossi A et al (1994) Unità di terapia intensiva respiratoria. Rassegna di patologia dell'apparato respiratorio 9(2):115–123

Cunnion RE, Natanson C (1994) Echocardiography, pulmonary artery catheterization, and radionuclide cineangiography in septic shock. Intensive Care Med 20(8):535–537

Ely WE, Inouye SK, Bernard GR et al (2001) Delirium in mechanically ventilated patients: validity and reliability of the confusion assessment method for the intensive care unit (CAM-ICU). JAMA 286(21):2703–2710

Grandjean T (1968) Une microtechnique du cathétérisme cardiaque droit praticable au lit du malade sans contrôle radioscopique (A microtechnic of right heart catheterization useful at the bedside without fluoroscopic monitoring). Cardiologie 51(3):184–192

Johnson DC, Batool S, Dalbec R (2008) Transcutaneous carbon dioxide pressure monitoring in a specialized weaning unit. Respir Care 53(8):1042–1047

Kelly BJ, Matthog MA (1993) Prevalence and severity of neurological dysfunction in critically ill patients. Influence on need for continued mechanical ventilation. Chest 104:1818–1824

Knaus WA, Draper EA, Wagner DP, Zimmerman JE (1985) APACHE II: a severity of disease classification system. Crit Care Med 13(10):18–23

Laghi F, Cattapan SE, Jubran A et al (2003) Is weaning failure caused by low-frequency fatigue of the diaphragm? Am J Respir Crit Care Med 167(2):120–127

Laporta D, Grassino A (1985) Assessment of transdiaphragmatic pressure in humans. J Appl Physiol 58(5):1469–1476

Lichtenstein DA, Meziére GA (2008) Relevance of lung ultrasound in the diagnosis of acute respiratory failure: the BLUE protocol. Chest 134(1):117–125

Lofaso F, Fodil R, Lorino H, Leroux K, Quintel A, Leroy A, Harf A (2000) Inaccuracy of tidal volume delivered by home mechanical ventilators. Eur Respir J 15(2):338–341

Milic-Emili J, Mead J, Turner JM, Glauser EM (1964) Improved technique for estimating pleural pressure from esophageal balloons. J Appl Physiol 19:207–211

Miller JM, Moxham J, Green M (1985) The maximal sniff in the assessment of diaphragm function in man. Clin Sci (Lond) 69(1):91–96

Nava S, Ambrosino N, Crotti P et al (1993) Recruitment of some respiratory muscles during three maximal inspiratory manoeuvres. Thorax 48(7):702–707

Sassoon CS, Te TT, Mahutte CK, Light RW (1987) Airway occlusion pressure. An important indicator for successful weaning in patients with chronic obstructive pulmonary disease. Am Rev Respir Dis 135(1):107–113

Talmor D, Sarge T, Malhotra A et al (2008) Mechanical ventilation guided by esophageal pressure in acute lung injury. N Engl J Med 359(20):2095–2104

Tobin MJ, Perez W, Guenther SM et al (1986) The pattern of breathing during successful and unsuccessful trials of weaning from mechanical ventilation. Am Rev Respir Dis 134(6):1111–1118

Tobin MJ (1988) Respiratory monitoring in the intensive care unit. Am Rev Respir Dis 138(6):1625–1642

Vassilakopoulos T (2008) Understanding wasted/ineffective efforts in mechanically ventilated COPD patients using the Campbell diagram. Intensive Care Med 34(7):1336–1339

Withelaw WA, Derenne JP, Milic-Emili J (1975) Occlusion pressure as a measure of respiratory center output in conscious man. Respir Physiol 23(2):181–199

Yang KL, Tobin MJ (1991) A prospective study of indexes predicting the outcome of trials of weaning from mechanical ventilation. N Engl J Med 324(21):1445–1450

How to Interpret the Curves on the Ventilator Screen

19

Our personal opinion, reached without the support of data meeting the criteria for evidence-based medicine, is that monitoring the flow, pressure and volume curves, at least in the first few hours of ventilation, is one of the keys to the success of NIV. The analysis of these signals in real time is particularly useful for evaluating the interaction between the patient and the machine.

The problem of synchrony during NIV is a particularly hot topic since we know that the inevitable presence of losses from the circuit is potentially associated with a poor interaction, unless the ventilator has very effective algorithms for compensation. The term synchrony derives from the combination of the Greek words $\sigma\iota\nu$ (*syn*, "with") and $\kappa\rho\rho\nu\rho\varsigma$ (*chronos*, "time") formally meaning a perfect correspondence between two signals. In this case, one talks of synchrony between the patient's timing and the ventilator's timing and, therefore, for example, of matching the patient's inspiratory time (Ti neural) and that of the ventilator (Ti vent). Physiology has taught us that the passage between the stimulus to breathing generated in the central nervous system and the contraction of the effector muscle is long and tortuous and that the electrical signal must precede the mechanical one.

That said, it is practically impossible to measure this delay in clinical practice, except in particular conditions, since only an electromyographic signal is able to record the neural Ti. A surrogate measurement of the electromyographic signal is a recording of the Pdi, remembering that the diaphragm can contract without there being a contemporaneous development of flow by the ventilator because of, for example, an intrinsic PEEP or a delay due to the algorithm for the inspiratory trigger. A Pdi recording is, however, a partially invasive technique, requiring specialist expertise; furthermore, it provides a fairly rough estimate of the electromyographic signal and is therefore susceptible to error.

The purpose of monitoring the curves on the ventilator screen is not, therefore, to measure time-related events precisely, such as the millisecond delay of the trigger, but rather more humbly to alert the clinician in the case of an evident dyssynchrony between the patient and the machine. Clinical determination of poor synchrony is not simply an intellectual game of interpreting signals; it is actually a clinically important alarm, since it has been extensively demonstrated that the

S. Nava and F. Fanfulla, *Non Invasive Artificial Ventilation*,
DOI: 10.1007/978-88-470-5526-1_19, © Springer-Verlag Italia 2014

presence of these changes can worsen clinical outcomes, for example, prolonging the duration of mechanical ventilation and thereby increasing the probability of requiring a tracheotomy.

Indeed, a recent study showed that the analysis of the waveforms generated by ventilators has a significant positive effect on physiological and patient-centered outcomes during acute exacerbation of COPD.

By examining the traces in the following figures we shall try to interpret the most obvious examples of poor matching.

Figure 19.1 represents the poor functioning of a ventilator trigger.

The flow trace clearly shows that the patient reaches the level of zero flow (end expiration) 360 ms before the ventilator is able to provide an inspiratory flow. That the patient has been able to reach the zero line means, by definition, that he has managed to overcome any intrinsic PEEP present, which we recall is the "useless" effort that the individual must make before reaching the equilibrium point of the respiratory system and before generating an inspiratory flow. Thus, simply from analyzing the flow signal, which takes on a plateau form immediately after having overcome the zero point, it is possible to identify a dyssynchrony, due in this case to poor functioning of the ventilator's algorithm, incorrect setting of the trigger, or mistaken assembly of the circuit.

Figure 19.2 shows one of the most frequent problems, that is, ineffective efforts, muscle contractions that are not able to trigger the ventilator. This phenomenon is particularly common in patients with obstructive disease who are ventilated at high inspiratory pressure since the high tidal volumes usually developed do not allow complete emptying of the air accumulated, and so the patient tries to stat a new breath when his degree of hyperinflation is too great to enable him to return to the equilibrium point of the respiratory system and, therefore, trigger the ventilator. Analysis of the flow parameters and airway pressures can reveal small, purposeless "bumps," which represent efforts that are not followed by, or are contemporaneous with, inspiratory support from the ventilator. These perturbations, particularly of the flow signal, suggest that the patient is trying to trigger the machine, but unsuccessfully.

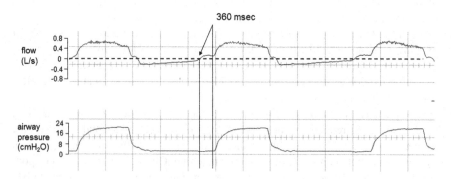

Fig. 19.1 How to recognize a delay in triggering

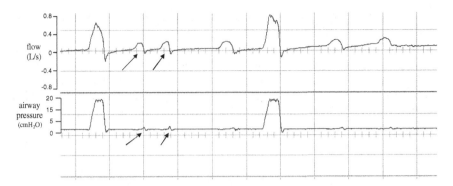

Fig. 19.2 Presence of ineffective efforts

Figure 19.3 shows a classic problem that is, in many cases, due to an incorrect setting by the operator. The presence of "doublets" or, as in this striking case, of "triplets" of flow and airway pressure suggests that there is a phenomenon called double-trigger, that is, an assisted inspiration followed very quickly (usually in less than 500 ms) by another. This phenomenon can be caused by a problem with the ventilator algorithm or the manual setting of too high an inspiratory flow and an overly sensitive expiratory trigger (that is, a trigger requiring only a very modest fall in peak flow, for example 20 %, to change from the inspiratory phase to the expiratory one).

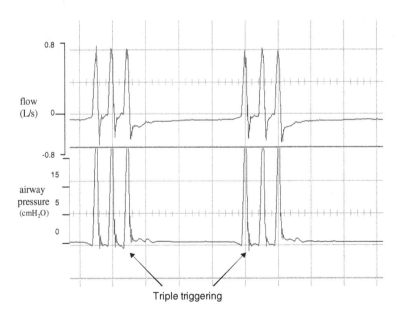

Triple triggering

Fig. 19.3 Presence of double or triple triggers

One classic problem of NIV is that of hang-up, which is an excessively prolonged inspiration caused by losses in the circuitry. In Fig. 19.4 the third breath has a longer inspiratory phase than the other breaths and the flow trace shows an initial fall followed by a plateau in a patient who does not seem to have reached the preestablished drop in flow in order to pass into the expiratory phase. The phenomenon of hang-up is almost always due to loss at the interface which interferes with the ventilator's algorithm responsible for regulating the change between inspiration and expiration which is performed, as in this case, when the inspiratory time is longer than the maximum established by default by the ventilator or by the operator.

The case of *auto-triggering*, that is, an inspiratory breath supported by the ventilator despite the patient not having made any demand, is not always easy to interpret since we do not usually have a Pdi trace, shown in Fig. 19.5. In the case of auto-triggering the Pdi trace remains "silent" although the patient receives inspiratory support. This can be due to the presence of an oversensitive inspiratory trigger or a disturbing factor, such as water in the circuit in the case of humidification by a heated humidifier.

There have been proposals for the use of algorithms for automatic, non invasive determination of gross problems with the patient/ventilator interaction, based on an analysis in real time of the flow and airway pressure signals. However, to our knowledge, no such algorithms have yet been incorporated in any ventilator.

Another piece of information that the flow curve can give us is a qualitative, but not quantitative, indication of the presence of intrinsic PEEP in the patient being ventilated. Typically the expiratory flow of a patient with dynamic hyperinflation and slowed emptying is characterized by the presence of expiratory flow until a few milliseconds before the start of the ventilatory support. As illustrated in Fig. 19.6, the trace shows a clear and sudden step that the flow makes, first to return to the zero line and then to become positive once the mechanical breath starts.

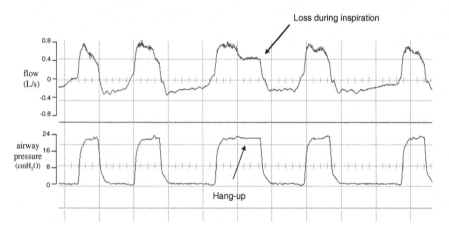

Fig. 19.4 The phenomenon of prolonged inspiration (hang-up) due to losses from the circuit

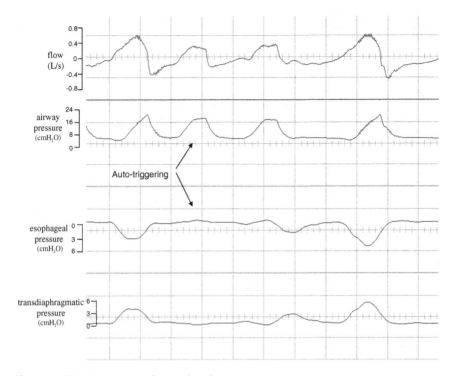

Fig. 19.5 The phenomenon of auto-triggering

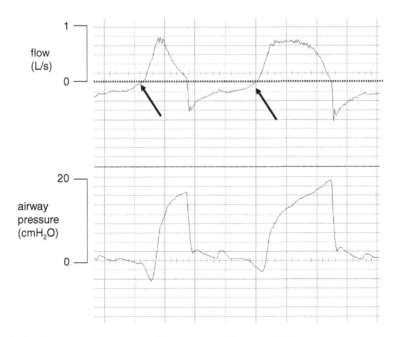

Fig. 19.6 How to recognize the possible presence of intrinsic PEEP

Suggested Reading

Calderini E, Confalonieri M, Puccio PG et al (1999) Patient–ventilator asynchrony during noninvasive ventilation: the role of expiratory trigger. Intensive Care Med 25(7):662–667

Carlucci A, Pisani L, Ceriana P, Malovini A, Nava S (2013) Patient–ventilator asynchronies: may the respiratory mechanics play a role? Crit Care 17:R54

Chao DC, Scheinhorn DJ, Stearn-Hassenpflug M (1997) Patient–ventilator trigger asynchrony in prolonged mechanical ventilation. Chest 112(6):1592–1599

Di Marco F, Centanni S, Bellone A, Messinesi G, Pesci A, Scala R, Perren A, Nava S (2011) Optimization of ventilator setting by flow and pressure waveforms analysis during noninvasive ventilation for acute exacerbations of COPD: a multicentric randomized controlled trial. Crit Care 15:R283

Hotchkiss JR, Adams AB, Dries DJ et al (2001) Dynamic behavior during noninvasive ventilation: chaotic support? Am J Respir Crit Care Med 163(2):374–378

Mulqueeny Q, Ceriana P, Carlucci A et al (2007) Automatic detection of ineffective triggering and double triggering during mechanical ventilation. Intensive Care Med 33(11):2014–2018

Nava S, Ceriana P (2005) Patient–ventilator interaction during noninvasive positive pressure ventilation. Respir Care Clin N Am 11(2):281–293

Nava S, Bruschi C, Rubini F et al (1995) Respiratory response and inspiratory effort during pressure support ventilation in COPD patients. Intensive Care Med 21(11):871–879

Nava S, Bruschi C, Fracchia C et al (1997) Patient–ventilator interaction and inspiratory effort during pressure support ventilation in patients with different pathologies. Eur Respir J 10(1):177–183

Ranieri VM, Giuliani R, Mascia L (1996) Patient–ventilator interaction during acute hypercapnia: pressure-support vs. proportional-assist ventilation. J Appl Physiol 81(1):426–436

Sassoon CS, Foster GT (2001) Patient–ventilator asynchrony. Curr Opin Crit Care 7(1):28–33

Thille AW, Rodriguez P, Cabello B (2006) Patient–ventilator asyncrony during assisted mechanical ventilation. Intensive Care Med 32(10):1515–1522

Vitacca M, Nava S, Confalonieri M et al (2000) The appropriate setting of noninvasive pressure support ventilation in stable COPD patients. Chest 118(5):1286–1293

Younes M, Brochard L, Grasso S et al (2007) A method for monitoring and improving patient: ventilator interaction. Intensive Care Med 33(8):1337–1346

Chronic Mechanical Ventilation: Is There a Rationale?

20

Chronic mechanical ventilation developed at the same time as modern acute mechanical ventilation. Already during the epidemic of poliomyelitis in the 1950s, it was clear that some patients would need chronic ventilatory support, whether partial or complete. At first, the only method of ventilation available for chronic use was intermittent negative pressure ventilation (NPV) via an iron lung. A care model was developed based on nocturnal sessions of ventilation therapy in hospital for those patients with some residual respiratory capacity or chronic hospitalization for those patients with no residual autonomy. It is clear that chronic ventilatory therapy, at home or not, was initially limited to those individuals who had an episode of acute respiratory failure and who, having survived, had become essentially ventilator-dependent. Subsequent scientific and technological progress enabled chronic home treatment for a large number of patients thanks to the production of smaller negative pressure ventilators ("poncho") and the development of intermittent positive pressure ventilators, initially used via a tracheostomy. The breakthrough in this sector arrived with the introduction of non invasive intermittent positive pressure ventilation, made possible by the availability of much smaller equipment.

A relatively recent investigation on home ventilation therapy in Europe, carried out between 2001 and 2002, collected extremely interesting information. First of all, it was possible to estimate the prevalence of such therapy, with 6.6/100,000 inhabitants undergoing chronic home ventilation treatment, equally distributed among the three groups of disorders considered (neuromuscular diseases, chest cage disorders and pathologies of the lung parenchyma). Thirteen percent of all the patients considered in this survey ($n = 21,526$) were being chronically ventilated via a tracheostomy, with the percentage differing according to the underlying disorder which had caused the chronic respiratory failure: the percentage was highest among patients with neuromuscular disorders (24 %) and lower in those with chronic parenchymal pathologies (8 %) or chest cage disorders (5 %).

There was a very marked variability in all the data from the different countries in Europe. Italy was distinguished by having the highest percentage of patients on home ventilation affected by pulmonary disorders (over 50 % of those being

S. Nava and F. Fanfulla, *Non Invasive Artificial Ventilation*,
DOI: 10.1007/978-88-470-5526-1_20, © Springer-Verlag Italia 2014

ventilated at home), greatly above the European mean (just over 30 %), and, together with Belgium, by the highest percentage of patients with lung disorders receiving chronic ventilation by an invasive route (about 20 % of all patients ventilated for these conditions). The European data demonstrate unequivocally that only a small minority of patients receiving chronic home ventilation treatment are doing so because of very severely limited or totally absent respiratory capacity, while there is extensive use in individuals with only partially compromised respiratory function.

What, therefore, is the rationale for using chronic ventilation in patients who still have some residual respiratory capacity? Essentially, three hypotheses have been proposed over the years, none of which excludes the others. These proposed mechanisms of action are summarized in Table 20.1.

The first hypothesis in order of time was that concerning the presence or possibility of chronic fatigue of the respiratory muscles; the idea was that allowing the muscles to rest periodically, for example during sleep, would improve their function. This hypothesis, proposed for patients affected by COPD, was based on the fact that numerous studies showed a marked reduction of electrical activity of the diaphragm during NIV and the observation that the maximum strength of the inspiratory muscles (MIP) improved after some sessions of NIV. However, two important aspects that limit the importance of these positive data do need to be highlighted: first, resting the respiratory muscles is not necessarily associated with an improvement in the chronic pump failure and second, the measurement of the MIP depends entirely on the patient's volition and is therefore susceptible to great

Table 20.1 Mechanisms of action of chronic non invasive mechanical ventilation in patients with chronic carbon dioxide retention

		Physiological principles
Main mechanisms	Rests respiratory muscles	Chronic weakness/fatigue of respiratory muscles
	Resets respiratory centers with ⇑ ventilatory response to CO_2 Reduces inspiratory resistances	Nocturnal alveolar hypoventilation
	Reduces $PEEP_i$. Improves lung volumes	Atelectasia, expiratory flow limitation, respiratory pattern
Secondary mechanisms		
	Improves sleep quality with ⇓ of daytime symptoms and ⇑ reactivity of respiratory centers	Sleep stabilization
	⇑Respiratory control	Restores circadian rhythm of control of respiration
	⇓Sympathetic tone	
	⇑ Quality of life	⇓ Plasma bicarbonate
	⇑ Efficacy of rehabilitation protocols	⇑ Exercise capacity

variability and a learning effect. A study by Schöenhofer et al. demonstrated that the improvements in clinical parameters and blood gases observed in a group of patients with severe hypercapnic chronic respiratory failure are not due to an increase in the strength of the respiratory muscles, evaluated in the study through measurement of transdiaphragmatic pressure elicited by bilateral stimuli of the phrenic nerve (2006). However, a state of weakness of the respiratory muscles is intrinsically present in patients with COPD as the result of the chronic overload that they must support. Indeed, Macgowan et al. showed that there were various structural alterations in the muscle fibers of the diaphragm, such as areas of necrosis, accumulation of lipofuscin, inflammatory infiltrates, and fibrosis and that the degree of these alterations was directly related to the severity of the bronchial obstruction (Macgowan et al. 2001) (Fig. 20.1) or hyperinflation (Gea et al. 2013). Intuitively, a state in which there are structural abnormalities of the respiratory muscles, such as during myopathies, will cause a progressive loss of muscle strength, thus promoting chronic retention of carbon dioxide.

The hypothesis that is currently most accredited is the correction of the state of hypoventilation during sleep that occurs in many disorders, in particular in those pathological conditions that respond to ventilation therapy. The pathological mechanisms that cause nocturnal alveolar hypoventilation are described in detail in the following chapters. Mechanical ventilation is thought to act directly on these mechanisms, correcting the clinical-functional consequences such as excessive daytime sleepiness, fatigue, diurnal hypercapnia, chronic cor polmonale, etc. It is thought that mechanical ventilation avoids accumulation of CO_2 during sleep, particularly during REM sleep, reducing the subsequent renal compensation through the increase of plasma bicarbonates, thereby enhancing the chemosensitivity of the respiratory centers. Intuitively, these positive effects could be obtained by administering ventilation therapy during sleep, but some studies have demonstrated that similar effects are also achieved with sessions of ventilation therapy limited only to the daytime hours. In any case, by reducing the accumulation of CO_2 during the night, nocturnal ventilation therapy gradually lowers the CO_2 levels during the day. In an elegant physiological study, Windisch and colleagues

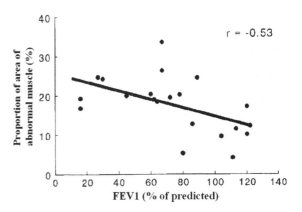

Fig. 20.1 Relationship between the proportion of cross-sectional area of altered diaphragmatic muscle fibers and severity of bronchial obstruction. Adapted from Macgowan et al. (2001), with permission from the American Thoracic Society, Official Journal of the American Thoracic Society©

(2006) observed, in two groups of patients with COPD and/or restrictive chest disorders, a progressive reduction in CO_2 in the first hours and a parallel increase in tidal volume during the daytime following sessions of nocturnal ventilation therapy, suggesting a clear improvement in responsiveness of the respiratory centers in the absence of significant changes in the strength of the respiratory muscles. Similar results had been obtained previously by Annane and colleagues (1999) in patients with neuromuscular disorders. On the other hand Karakurt and colleagues, analyzing the changes in blood gases and respiratory pattern that occurred during the day in a group of patients after acute withdrawal of their chronic, showed that the patients who had to restart ventilation early were those who had the greatest change in $PaCO_2$ between spontaneous breathing and mechanical ventilation and a higher mean inspiratory flow during spontaneous respiration—in other words, the patients with the greatest respiratory muscle impairment and the greatest activation of central respiratory drive.

The third hypothesis is based on changes in the mechanical properties of the respiratory system induced by chronic mechanical ventilation therapy. Some studies carried out in patients with neuromuscular disorders showed an increase in vital capacity after prolonged treatment with NIV. The mechanism of this change is suggested to be related to an improvement in compliance as a result of the anticipated collapse of the small airways and a reduction in microatelectasia (Fig. 20.2). In contrast, in patients affected by COPD it was demonstrated that the improvement in blood gases seen during non invasive mechanical ventilation is related to the reduction in the degree of alveolar hyperinflation and inspiratory load, and a deeper, slower respiratory pattern. In fact, it has been shown that PEEPi is present, to a variable degree but in any case less than during exacerbations, in patients with COPD who are clinically and functionally stable.

The application of CPAP seems to have a minimal effect on inspiratory load, at least if the level of CPAP applied is higher than the level of measured PEEPi, as reported by O'Donoghue et al. (2002). This strategy led to a significant reduction

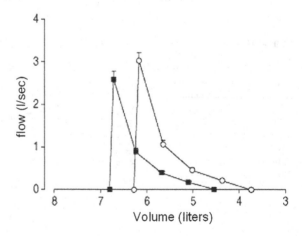

Fig. 20.2 Maximal expiratory flow/volume curves at baseline (*black squares*) and after 3 weeks of non invasive mechanical ventilation (*white circles*). Adapted from Diaz et al. Eur Respir J 2002 with permission from European Respiratory Society Journals Ltd

in the indices of inspiratory muscle strength together with a substantial increase in lung volumes. The reduction in inspiratory effort seemed to be out of proportion to the elastic load (PEEPi) present, so other mechanisms of action of CPAP have been hypothesized: a reduction in the resistance of the upper and lower airways, decreased distortion of the chest cage, and stabilization of the small airways with improvement of lung compliance (McKenzie et al. 2009).

Other minor effects of the use of non invasive mechanical ventilation are summarized in Table 20.1. These are related to improvements in sleep, quality of life, functional state, response to rehabilitation treatment, exercise capacity as measured by the 6-min walking test, recovery of normal circadian modulation of respiratory rhythm, and a reduction in sympathetic tone.

Suggested Reading

Annane D, Quera-Salva MA, Lofaso F et al (1999) Mechanisms underlying effects of nocturnal ventilation on daytime blood gases in neuromuscular diseases. Eur Respir J 13(1):157–162

Baydur A, Layne E, Aral H et al (2000) Long term non-invasive ventilation in the community for patients with musculoskeletal disorders: 46 years experience and review. Thorax 55(1):4–11

Dìaz O, Bégin P, Torrealba B et al (2002) Effects of noninvasive ventilation on lung hyperinflation in stable hypercapnic COPD. Eur Respir J 20(6):1490–1498

Dìaz O, Bégin P, Andresen M et al (2005) Physiological and clinical effects of diurnal noninvasive ventilation in hypercapnic COPD. Eur Respir J 26(6):1016–1023

Duiverman ML, Bladder G, Meinesz AF, Wijkstra PJ (2006) Home mechanical ventilatory support in patients with restrictive ventilatory disorders: a 48-year experience. Respir Med 100(1):56–65

Duiverman DL, Wempe JB, Bladder G et al (2008) Nocturnal non-invasive ventilation in addition to rehabilitation in hypercapnic patients with COPD. Thorax 63(12):1052–1057

Gea J, Agustì A, Roca J (2013) Pathophysiology of muscle dysfuntion in COPD. J Appl Physiol 114:1222–1234

Karakurt S, Fanfulla F, Nava S (2001) Is it safe for patients with chronic hypercapnic respiratory failure undergoing home non-invasive ventilation to discontinue ventilation briefly? Chest 119:1379–1386

Lloyd-Owen SJ, Donaldson GC, Ambrosino N et al (2005) Patterns of home mechanical ventilation use in Europe: results from the eurovent survey. Eur Respir J 25(6):1025–1031

Macgowan NA, Evans KG, Road JD, Reid WD (2001) Diaphragm injury in individuals with airflow obstruction. Am J Respir Crit Care Med 163(7):1654–1659

McKenzie DK, Butler JE, Gandevia SC (2009) Respiratory muscle function and activation in chronic obstructive pulmonary disease. J Appl Physiol 107:621–629

O'Donoghue FJ, Catcheside PG, Jordan AS et al (2002) Effect of CPAP on intrinsic PEEP, inspiratory effort, and lung volume in severe stable COPD. Thorax 57(6):533–539

Schöenhofer B, Polkey MI, Suchi S, Köhler D (2006) Effect of home mechanical ventilation on inspiratory muscle strenght in COPD. Chest 130(6):1834–1838

Sin DD, Wong E, Mayers I et al (2007) Effects of nocturnal noninvasive mechanical ventilation on heart rate variability of patients with advanced COPD. Chest 131(1):156–163

Spengler CM, Czeisler CA, Shea SA (2000) An endogenous circadian rhythm of respiratory control in humans. J Physiol 526(Pt 3):683–694

Windisch W, Dreher M, Storre JH, Sorichter S (2006) Nocturnal non-invasive positive pressure ventilation: physiological effects on spontaneous breathing. Respir Physiol Neurobiol 150(2–3):251–260

Chronic Ventilation in COPD

21

Chronic obstructive pulmonary disease (COPD) is a progressive, irreversible disorder that usually leads to the development of chronic respiratory failure.

It is one of the main causes of death from chronic disease in the world. Its high prevalence associated with the increase in mean life expectancy in more affluent countries are the two factors that have made this disease one of the major causes of healthcare expenditure.

In its advanced stages, especially after the development of a state of chronic respiratory failure, and despite optimization of pharmacological therapy, COPD is characterized by symptoms that limit normal daily life activities and quality of life, and by frequent exacerbations which often culminate in admission to hospital. A high percentage of patients discharged from a hospital after an admission for an exacerbation of COPD will be readmitted within a year for another similar episode.

The only therapeutic intervention that has been demonstrated to be effective in improving the survival of patients with COPD and severe daytime hypoxemia is long-term oxygen therapy (LTOT). For this reason, the healthcare systems in numerous countries have allocated specific funds to finance home oxygen therapy for all those patients requiring LTOT.

Various studies have demonstrated that integrated rehabilitation treatment is able to improve dyspnea, exercise tolerance, and quality of life even in patients already in chronic respiratory failure. The possible therapeutic interventions for patients with COPD are reported in Table 21.1. Despite this, the life expectancy of patients with COPD who are receiving LTOT for chronic respiratory failure is reduced, with a 5-year survival rate of about 40 %. Various factors negatively affect the prognosis of these patients: spirometric indices, reduced carbon monoxide transfer, severity of the hypoxemia and hypercapnia, reduced exercise capacity, degree of dyspnea, body mass, general state of health, and number of exacerbations per year.

As mentioned above, exacerbations are the most frequent cause of hospital admissions and are associated with a fairly high mortality rate; about 10 % considering a single admission and up to 40 % within the year following the acute

Table 21.1 Therapeutic options for patients with COPD

	Indications	Type of intervention
Pharmacological treatment	Symptomatic patients with FEV_1 <60 % of predicted	• Inhaled long-acting β_2-agonists
		• Inhaled long-acting anticholinergic drugs
		• Inhaled steroids: alone or in combination
Long-term oxygen therapy	• Stable hypoxemia (PaO_2 < 55 mmHg)	Stabilize SaO_2 > 92 %
	• Nocturnal hypoxemia	
	• Hypoxemia during physical activity	
Pulmonary rehabilitation	Patients with moderate-severe COPD with or without respiratory failure	• Physical exercise or endurance training
		• Educational sessions
		• Behavioral therapy
		• Training of respiratory muscles
		• Training of upper/ lower limbs

admission. Furthermore, the rate of repeated admissions to hospital is high among these patients; one epidemiological study showed that 63 % of patients with COPD who required LTOT were readmitted to hospital during a mean follow-up period of 1.1 years.

Various healthcare programs, mostly multidisciplinary, have been developed in different countries to ensure adequate continuity of care for patients with progressive chronic diseases with the aims of improving control of the disease, reducing hospital admissions, and lowering the mortality rate. Conflicting results have been obtained; only programs specifically designed for patients with COPD have shown a good efficacy, especially when the protocol includes specific rehabilitation interventions.

The use of non invasive mechanical ventilation in patients with COPD and chronic respiratory failure is still scientifically controversial. However, an epidemiological study carried out in Europe on prescriptions of non invasive home ventilation therapy, which involved 239 centers and 21,526 patients, showed that COPD is one of the main indications for this treatment. It could, therefore, be concluded that, despite the lack of unequivocal scientific evidence and/or definitive criteria for its prescription and method of application, clinicians have been able to identify reasons for its chronic use in individual patients. Indeed, patients with very advanced COPD usually have a relevant degree of alveolar hyperinflation that worsens the mechanical respiratory load considerably and leads to reduced function of the respiratory muscles, in particular the diaphragm. Chronic hyperinflation causes a flattening of the diaphragm, reducing the length of the sarcomeres and, therefore, the capacity to generate force since the muscle works in a disadvantageous part of the tension–length curve. In addition, the reduced area of apposition between the diaphragm and the chest cage further limits the pumping capacity of the main respiratory muscle.

The main consequence of these functional limitations is recruitment of the accessory inspiratory muscles, which causes an increase in oxygen consumption necessary to guarantee sufficient respiratory activity. Chronic submaximal activation of all the inspiratory muscles reduces their functional reserve, contributing to a further worsening in the already compromised capacity to carry out physical activity and increasing the risk of muscle fatigue. Positive pressure NIV gives the chronically activated muscles periods of rest, thereby promoting a partial recovery of their strength and resistance. At the same time, the use of chronic NIV during the night can correct episodes of hypoventilation during sleep, thereby improving sleep quality, function of the respiratory centers, and, finally, gas exchange while awake. All the possible positive effects of chronic ventilation therapy are summarized in Fig. 21.1.

Despite the premises above and the widespread use of this treatment in daily clinical practice, as of yet few studies have been performed with the purpose of evaluating the effect of chronic ventilation treatment in patients with COPD and chronic respiratory failure and those that have been performed are very heterogeneous. The limited data available have been the subject of repeated reviews and meta-analyses, all of which concordantly conclude that this treatment can have a

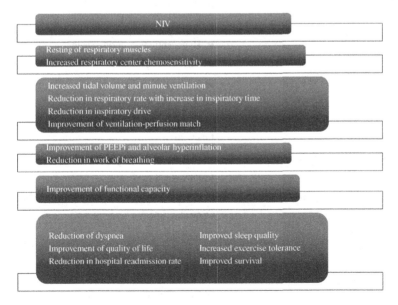

Fig. 21.1 Possible effects of long-term NIV in patients with COPD and hypercapnic chronic respiratory failure. All the effects listed have been demonstrated in published studies

role in selected patients and that further studies are necessary to identify the most appropriate candidates and define the expected outcomes. There are numerous explanations for the lack of definitive data, but probably the difficulty in recruiting a sufficient number of patients and the need to monitor them for a long time, which requires a very complex and multicenter organization, have limited the possibility of carrying out large clinical trials. The studies performed so far have had very substantial differences, as summarized in Table 21.2. In the first place, they were published over a period of about 20 years; it is objectively difficult to compare studies designed and carried out in the 1980s with similar studies performed recently.

Another characteristic that emerges, particularly in the older studies, is the high percentage of drop-outs. It has been known for some time that NIV is less well tolerated by patients with COPD than by those with a restrictive disease, but a precise explanation for this has not yet been found. One appealing hypothesis is that the adherence to treatment depends on the type of ventilation applied. Finally, another important aspect that further complicates the comparison of the data in the

Table 21.2 Main methodological differences between published studies that evaluated the efficacy of NIV therapy in COPD patients in a clinically stable condition

Experimental design	✔ RCT/non-RCT—Cross-over
	✔ Duration of follow-up- Statistical analysis
	✔ Sample size—Drop-out rate
Clinical physiological characteristics of the patients	✔ Bronchial obstruction
	✔ Blood-gases
	✔ Respiratory muscle weakness
	✔ Hypoventilation during sleep
Physiological outcome measures	✔ Gas exchange
	✔ Spirometric indices
	✔ Respiratory pattern
	✔ Respiratory mechanics (respiratory work/muscle function)
Clinical outcome measures	✔ Improvement of dyspnea
	✔ Functional state
	✔ Tolerance of physical exercise
	✔ Quality of life
	✔ Morbidity
	✔ Mortality
	✔ Compliance
Ventilation	✔ Type of mechanical ventilation
	✔ Setting of the ventilator parameters

literature is the duration of the follow-up, which varies from less than 1 week to 5 years. Consequently, here we limit ourselves to analyzing some of most important studies published in the literature.

In 1991, Strumpf and colleagues published the results of a study of 19 patients with COPD and $FEV_1 < 1$ L, of whom 12 withdrew from the study for the following reasons: seven were unable to tolerate the mask and five developed another disease. Only three of the seven ventilated patients reported an improvement in their dyspnea during ventilation; however, analysis of the respiratory function tests, maximal inspiratory pressure, blood-gas exchange, exercise capacity and sleep architecture, and efficiency did not show any improvement over conventional therapy. The single significant effect was observed in neuropsychological function, and was probably related to a placebo effect. Despite the limited number of patients, the authors concluded that patients with COPD did not tolerate nocturnal NIV well and that this type of ventilation did not lead to any clinical improvement in the patients. It should, however, be pointed out that the subjects enrolled were fairly atypical, being formed of patients with modest hypoxemia and blood CO_2 levels essentially within the norm ($PaCO_2$ at enrollment = 46 ± 2 mmHg) (Strumpf et al. 1991).

Subsequently, Meecham Jones and colleagues studied 18 clinically stable patients with hypoxia (mean $PaO_2 = 45.3$ mmHg) and hypercapnia (mean $PaCO_2 = 55.8$ mmHg). Fourteen of these patients completed the 3-month study, and only one was excluded because of ventilator intolerance (Meecham Jones et al. 1995). The randomized, cross-over design of the study was intended to compare NIV + LTOT versus oxygen therapy alone. The authors observed a significant improvement due to NIV with regards to diurnal gas exchange, total sleep time, sleep efficiency, and $PaCO_2$ recorded during the night, as well as quality of life assessed using the St. George's questionnaire. The improvement in daytime $PaCO_2$ was significantly related to the decrease in nocturnal $PaCO_2$ (Fig. 21.2). The conclusion, which contrasted with that of the North American study, was,

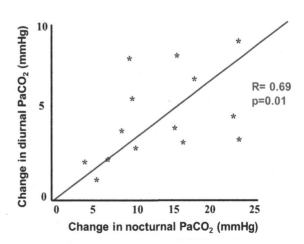

Fig. 21.2 Relationship between nocturnal and diurnal carbon dioxide levels after starting ventilation therapy. Modified from Meecham Jones et al. (1995), with permission from the American Thoracic Society, official journal of the American Thoracic Society©

R= 0.69
p=0.01

therefore, that NIV could be useful in combination with oxygen therapy in the treatment of stable, hypercapnic COPD.

The contradiction between the results of the two studies can be explained, at least in part. The methods of ventilation used were fairly different in the two studies: BiPAP in spontaneous mode, used in the study by Meecham Jones, probably enables a better patient–ventilator interaction compared to the timed mode, used by Strumpf, in which the patient is forced to follow the rhythm of the ventilator. It is interesting to note that in Strumpf's study the patients spent at least 25 % of the night in asynchrony with the ventilator. Another interesting aspect is the different levels of CO_2 in the patients enrolled. It is known from studies of acute care that hypercapnic patients respond better than normocapnic patients to trials of NIV and this could also hold true for chronic treatment, as seen in studies by Carroll and by Marino in which the patients who adapted successfully to ventilation belonged to this subgroup.

A subsequent randomized, controlled trial carried out by Casanova et al. enrolled 52 patients with severe, but stable, COPD; 44 completed the 12 months of follow-up. The aim of the study was to evaluate the efficacy of nocturnal NIV compared to standard, conventional treatment. The outcome parameters were the level of dyspnea, blood-gases during spontaneous breathing, respiratory and neuropsychological function, hematological and hemodynamic parameters, morbidity (exacerbations, intubation rate, hospital admissions) and mortality. The authors concluded that NIV did not alter the natural history of COPD and that its benefits are only marginal in patients with clinically stable COPD. In fact, no significant differences were seen in either mortality or morbidity and the only benefits observed were in the degree of dyspnea (measured using Borg's scale) and in one neuropsychological test (psychomotor coordination). However, this study was open to numerous criticisms, the most important of which was the number of patients with regards to the outcomes studied (52 patients, 26 per arm, for six categories of outcomes!). In fact, the size of the study population was calculated only taking into account a possible difference of 10 % compared to the expected mortality rate. Furthermore, some of the patients enrolled were not hypercapnic or did not even require LTOT (in other words, they did not have respiratory failure). Finally, the settings of the ventilation therapy were based on the efficacy measure of a visual reduction in the use of accessory muscles, a reduction in the perception of dyspnea and a 20 % decrease in respiratory rate. In other words, there was no objective measurement of the ventilation therapy either during the period awake or during sleep, this latter being particularly important considering that this was a ventilation therapy to be administered during sleep.

These results are in clear contrast to those subsequently obtained in a study carried out by the Italian Association of Pulmonologists and published in 2002, which involved a group of patients with COPD and chronic hypercapnic respiratory failure ($PaCO_2$ at enrollment >50 mmHg with pH > 7.35) receiving LTOT for at least 6 months (Clini et al. 2002). The aim of this study, the first to extend the follow-up to 2 years, was to establish the effects of NIV combined with LTOT on the severity of hypercapnia, use of healthcare resources and quality of life, comparing them with the effects in a randomized control group of patients who received only standard treatment and LTOT. One hundred and twenty-two patients were enrolled, of whom 86 were randomized; 47 patients completed the study, 16 died (8 in each arm), and 23 dropped out. The primary outcomes were blood-gases, hospital admissions, and admissions to an intensive care unit, duration of the admissions, and quality of life measures; secondary outcomes were survival, drop-out rate, symptoms, and exercise tolerance. The clearest results were the reductions in blood CO_2 level recorded during the oxygen therapy (Fig. 21.3a) and level of dyspnea at rest (Fig. 21.3b) and the improvement in quality of life. Furthermore, compared to the period preceding the study, the authors noted a clear trend to a reduction of hospital admissions (-45 % in the NIV group compared to $+27$ % in the LTOT group) and admissions to intensive care units (-75 % in the NIV group compared to -20 % in the LTOT group); unfortunately, these differences did not reach statistical significance. No difference was seen in mortality between the two groups.

The first study, albeit not randomized, which found a reduction in mortality rate in patients with COPD undergoing chronic ventilation therapy was published by Budweiser and colleagues in 2007 (Budweiser et al. 2007). In a 4-year follow-up, the authors compared the survival curves of 140 patients with severe, persistent hypercapnia ($PaCO_2$ 60.1 ± 9.2 mmHg) who received NIV ($n = 99$) or did not receive NIV ($n = 41$). The adherence to the ventilation therapy was very high (88.9 %) with a daily use of 6.4 ± 2.6 h. The 1- and 2-year survival rates in

Fig. 21.3 Changes in blood carbon dioxide levels during oxygen treatment (**a**) and degree of dyspnea at rest (**b**) in patients undergoing NIV and LTOT compared to those in patients receiving only LTOT: *Black diamonds* Long-term oxygen therapy; *Black circles* NIV and long-term oxygen therapy. Adapted from Clini et al. (2002), with permission from the European Respiratory Society Journals Ltd

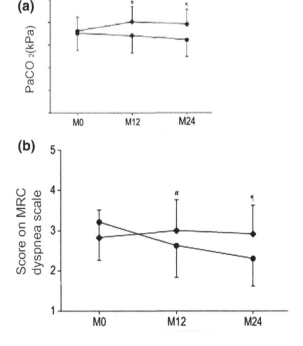

patients undergoing NIV were 87.7 and 71.8 %, respectively, whereas the corresponding figures for patients receiving standard therapy were 56.7 and 42.0 %, respectively.

In a subsequent analysis stratified by risk factors the authors showed that the benefit was greatest in some groups of patients, such as those with a higher base excess (BE > 8.9 mmol/L), lower pH values (<7.41), lower FEV_1 (<27.5 %), lower hemoglobin (<13.8 g/dL), or greater alveolar hyperinflation (Motley index > 189 % of predicted). Although this was an observational study, it is important not only because it was the first to demonstrate an effect of NIV on survival rate, but also because it seemed to identify subgroups of patients in whom this effect is greater.

The improvement in survival was further confirmed in an important Australian study published in 2009; at last, there was a randomized, controlled trial with a flawless design, and exemplary statistics (McEvoy et al. 2009). The study (the AVCAL study) was carried out between 1998 and 2004 in four university hospitals in Australia in patients with severe COPD and hypercapnic chronic respiratory failure ($PaCO_2 > 46$ mmHg) who had received LTOT for at least 3 months and who were clinically stable; the aim was to evaluate the effects of NIV on survival, lung function, and quality of life compared to the effects of standard LTOT. The enrollment of the patients was particularly challenging, as it was in the AIPO study, demonstrating the difficulty in conducting this type of research; in the end, 144 patients were randomized, 72 per arm. The results were particularly important even if of mixed significance. In the first place, NIV significantly improved sleep quality and the related hypercapnia acutely in all patients, whereas during the follow-up it had these effects only in the patients with good adherence to treatment. Furthermore, NIV increased the survival rate (in the intention-to-treat analysis), although this was statistically significant only after adjusting for confounding factors (hazard ratio 0.63, $p = 0.045$) (Fig. 21.4). However, the improvement in survival rate appeared greater in patients with better adherence to the ventilation therapy who used this treatment for more than 4 h/night (hazard ratio 0.57, $p = 0.036$). Quality of life parameters, measured using the disease-specific St. George's questionnaire, were not different between the two groups of patients considered. Surprisingly, patients being treated with NIV had worse scores in some dimensions of the Short Form-36 (SF-36), a questionnaire that measures quality of life and mood; thus patients undergoing NIV reported a worse quality of life. This was in contrast to the findings of the Italian study which had similar enrollment criteria. The Italian study used the MRF-28 questionnaire (Maugeri Foundation Respiratory Failure Questionnaire) (Carone et al. 1999), which is a more sensitive and specific assessment of quality of life than that afforded by the St. George's questionnaire (Jones et al. 1992) in patients with chronic respiratory failure. The authors ascribed the worsening mood in patients undergoing NIV to the complexity of the treatment without perceptible improvements, from the patient's point of view, in health status. An alternative hypothesis highlighted by the same authors is the possibility of a "survival effect;" worsening mood would be due to increasing severity of the disease, made possible by the longer survival.

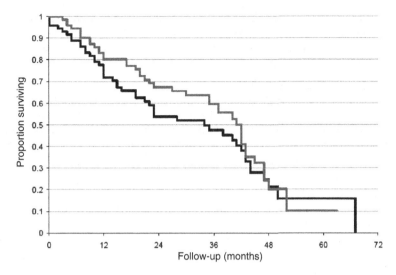

Fig. 21.4 Survival curves of patients undergoing NIV and patients in a control group. *Dark line*: patients receiving LTOT; *Pale line*: patients receiving NIV and LTOT. Adapted from McEvoy et al. (2009), with permission from the BMJ Publishing Group Ltd

21.1   Indications for Prescribing NIV and Possible Outcomes

As we have seen, the current scientific evidence does not unequivocally support the use of NIV in patients with COPD. Nonetheless, it is worth repeating that this therapeutic option is widely used by clinicians every day, especially in Italy. Its routine use is based on the indications set out in international consensus statements or guidelines from scientific societies, which are evidently more oriented to a clinical approach.

The presence of a state of chronic, severe hypercapnia ($PaCO_2 > 55$ mmHg), with associated symptoms, can be considered one of the major criteria for evaluating whether to start long-term ventilation therapy; another criterion is the impossibility of weaning a patient from ventilation therapy, even NIV, after an episode of acute respiratory failure.

Alternatively, this treatment is often used in patients with lower $PaCO_2$ values (range, 50–55 mmHg) but with signs and symptoms of alveolar hypoventilation during sleep, despite the use of optimized oxygen therapy. The indication for home NIV was proposed in the International Consensus Conference on the indications for intermittent positive pressure NIV in patients with chronic respiratory failure, the proceedings of which were published in Chest in 1999 (Consensus Conference 1999). These indications have remained substantially valid and were subsequently repeated in the GOLD guidelines, which suggest the use of home NIV in patients with pronounced daytime hypercapnia (Vestbo et al. 2013).

Another indication for long-term NIV is frequent episodes (at least two in the arc of 12 months) of hypercapnic respiratory failure requiring admission to hospital. Various studies have documented that long-term NIV lowers the rate of hospital admissions for acidotic exacerbations in patients with COPD, with consequent improvement in survival and a not irrelevant reduction in costs of the management of this disorder, particularly due to the net decrease in admissions to an intensive care unit. Indeed, in a study by Tuggey and colleagues, carried out in the UK, it was calculated that more than €10,000/year/patient was saved after starting ventilation therapy, although it should be noted that the patients enrolled in this study were highly selected (Tuggey et al. 2003). This finding was subsequently confirmed by Clini and colleagues in their analysis of the data from a multicenter Italian study (Clini et al. 2009).

The indications for chronic ventilation therapy proposed by the International Consensus Conference are summarized in Fig. 21.4. These indications generally concern very severely ill patients whose life expectancy is greatly reduced. In fact, in a recent 10-year follow-up study which compared two methods of management of patients with chronic respiratory failure due to COPD being treated with LTOT, Rizzi, and colleagues demonstrated that the need to start long-term NIV, according to the indications of the Consensus Conference, is an independent predictor of mortality. The mean survival of patients undergoing NIV was 10.9 months (standard deviation 4.9 months). In a prospective study, Budweiser and colleagues investigated the strongest predictors of mortality in patients with hypercapnic chronic respiratory failure receiving long-term NIV (Budweiser et al. 2007). The criteria used for starting NIV were the presence of hypercapnia permanently above 50 mmHg together with chronic symptoms or, alternatively, $PaCO_2$ permanently above 45 mmHg together with repeated episodes of acute hypercapnic respiratory failure, dyspnea at rest, or severely compromised lung function. The overall mortality rate was 44.7 %, while the survival rates at 1, 2 and 5 years were 84, 65.3, and 26.4 %, respectively. Multivariate analysis showed that, among all parameters recorded at enrollment, significant predictors of mortality were age, body mass index (BMI), Motley's index (residual volume/total lung capacity), and the level of the base excess. However, the most interesting finding was the prognostic value of changes in some functional indices observed after the start of ventilation therapy. The changes that were found to be associated with an improvement in prognosis were an increase in BMI in patients with a baseline BMI <25 kg/m^2, a reduction of at least 4 % in Motley's index in patients with a baseline score of ≥73 %, and a 50 % reduction in the base excess in patients who, at enrollment, had a value ≥9 mmol/L.

Are there margins for the use of NIV in patients with less severe disease? The initial study by Meecham Jones and the more recent Australian one, the AVCAL study, showed significant clinical and functional improvements, as well as a better survival, when the main indication was the correction of nocturnal alveolar hypoventilation (Meecham Jones et al. 1995; McEvoy et al. 2009). Other interesting indications concern the use of NIV in combination with classical rehabilitation programs. Indeed, Duiverman and colleagues showed that nocturnal NIV enhanced the positive effects of pulmonary rehabilitation in patients with hypercapnic chronic respiratory failure (Duiverman et al. 2008). The authors enrolled 72 patients, divided into two groups according to a random sequence: the patients in one group underwent a multidisciplinary program of respiratory rehabilitation lasting 12 weeks, while the other group received nocturnal ventilation therapy in addition to the same rehabilitation program as that used in the first group. At the end of the therapeutic program, the patients who had undergone rehabilitation treatment combined with NIV had improved blood CO_2 levels during both the night and the day, improved quality of life from various points of view, and an increase in daily physical activity, expressed as the number of steps taken during a day. These results were confirmed after a 2-year follow-up (Duiverman et al. 2011).

21.2   Conclusions

At present, advanced COPD cannot be considered a systematic therapeutic option in patients with hypercapnic respiratory failure. Although the most recent scientific evidence does seem to open up interesting perspectives for survival, improved quality of life, and greater functional efficacy, much still remains to be understood, particularly with regards to identifying the best candidates for this therapy. Future research could clarify which indices of respiratory function (breathing control, respiratory work, muscle strength, blood-gases, acid-base balance), both during sleep and while awake, and which neuropsychological features, settings and modes of ventilation or modes of home care could become parameters for identifying the most suitable candidates for this specific type of complex treatment.

Suggested Reading

Annane D, Chevrolet JC, Chevret S, Raphael JC (2000) Nocturnal mechanical ventilation for chronic hypoventilation in patients with neuromuscular and chest wall disorders. Cochrane Database Syst Rev 4(2):CD001941. doi:10.1002/14651858.CD001941.pub2

Budweiser S, Jörres RA, Riedl T et al (2007) Predictors of survival in COPD patients with chronic hypercapnic respiratory failure receiving noninvasive home ventilation. Chest 131(6):1650–1658

Carone M, Bertolotti G, Anchisi F et al (1999) Analysis of factors that characterize health impairment in patients with chronic respiratory failure. Eur Respir J 13(6):1293–1300 (Quality of Life in Chronic Respiratory Failure Group)

Carroll N, Branthwaithe MA (1988) Control of nocturnal hypoventilation by nasal IPPV. Thorax 43:349–353

Casanova C, Celli BR, Tost L et al (2000) Long-term controlled trial of nocturnal nasal positive pressure ventilation patients with severe COPD. Chest 118(6):1582–1590

Celli BR, Cote CG, Marin JM et al (2004) The body-mass index, airflow obstruction, dyspnea, and exercise capacity index in chronic obstructive pulmonary disease. N Engl J Med 350(10):1005–1012

Clini E, Sturani C, Rossi A et al (2002) The Italian multicentre study on noninvasive ventilation in chronic obstructive pulmonary disease patients. Eur Respir J 20(3):529–538 [Rehabilitation and Chronic Care Study Group, Italian Association of Hospital Pulmonologists (AIPO)]

Clini EM, Magni G, Crisafulli E et al (2009) Home non-invasive mechanical ventilation and long-term oxygen therapy in stable hypercapnic chronic obstructive pulmonary disease patients: comparison of costs. Respiration 77(1):44–50

Connors AF Jr, Dawson NV, Thomas C et al (1996) Outcomes following acute exacerbation of severe chronic obstructive lung disease. Am J Respir Crit Care Med 154(4):959–967 [The SUPPORT investigators (Study to Understand Prognoses and Preferences for Outcomes and Risks of Treatment)]

Duiverman ML, Wempe JB, Bladder G et al (2008) Nocturnal non-invasive ventilation in addition to rehabilitation in hypercapnic patients with COPD. Thorax 63(12):1052–1057

Duiverman ML, Wempe JB, Bladder G et al (2011) Two-year home-based nocturnal noninvasive ventilation added to rehabilitation in chornic obstructive pulmonary disease patients: a randomized controlled trial. Respir Res 12:112

Elliott MW, Steven MH, Phillips GD, Branthwaite MA (1990) Non-invasive mechanical ventilation for acute respriratory failure. BMJ 300(6721):358–360

Elliott MW, Mulvey DA, Moxham J et al (1991) Domiciliary nocturnal nasal intermittent positive pressure ventilation in COPD: mechanisms underlying changes in arterial blood gas tensions. Eur Respir J 4(9):1044–1052

Funk GC, Breyer MK, Burghuber OC et al (2011) Long-term non-invasive ventilation in COPD after acute-on-chronic respiratory failure. Respir Med 105:427–434

Funk GC, Bauer P, Burghuber OC et al (2012) Prevalence and prognosis of chronic obstructive pulmonary disease in critically ill patients between 1998 and 2008. ERJ 41:792–799

Garcia-Aymerich J, Farrero E, Félez MA et al (2003) Risk factors of readmission to hospital for a COPD exacerbation: a prospective study. Thorax 58(2):100–105

Gay PC, Hubmayr RD, Stroetz RW (1996) Efficacy of nocturnal nasal ventilation in stable, severe chronic obstructive pulmonary disease during a 3-month controlled trial. Mayo Clin Proc 71(6):533–542

Kvale PA (1999) Clinical indications for noninvasive positive pressure ventilation in chronic respiratory failure due to restrictive lung disease, COPD, and nocturnal hypoventilation—a consensus conference report. Chest 116(2):521–535

(2011) Global initiative for chronic obstructive lung disease. Workshop report, global strategy for diagnosis, management, and prevention of COPD. Revised 2011. Available from www.goldcopd.com

Groenewegen KH, Schols AM, Wouters EF (2003) Mortality and mortality-related factors after hospitalization for acute exacerbation of COPD. Chest 124(2):459–467

Gunen H, Hacievliyagil SS, Kosar F et al (2005) Factors affecting survival of hospitalised patients with COPD. Eur Respir J 26(2):234–241

Heinemann F, Budweiser S, Jörres RA, Arzt M, Rösch F, Kollert F, Pfeifer M (2011) The role of non-invasive home mechanical ventilation in patients with chronic obstructive pulmonary disease requiring prolonged weaning. Respirology 16:1273–1280

Jones PW, Quirk FH, Baveystock CM, Littlejohns P (1992) A self-complete measure of health status for chronic airflow limitation: the St. George's Respiratory Questionnaire. Am Rev Respir Dis 145(6):1321–1327

Jones SE, Packham S, Hebden M, Smith AP (1998) Domiciliary nocturnal intermittent positive pressure ventilation in patients with respiratory failure due to severe COPD: long-term follow up and effect on survival. Thorax 53(6):495–498

Kolodziej MA, Jensen L, Rowe B, Sin D (2007) Systematic review of noninvasive positive pressure ventilation in severe stable COPD. Eur Respir J 30(2):293–306

Loddenkemper R, Gibson GJ, Sibille Y (2003) European Lung White Book: the first comprehensive survey on respiratory heath in Europe. European Respiratory Society, Sheffield

Machado MC, Krishnan JA, Buist SA et al (2006) Sex differences in survival of oxygen-dependent patients with chronic obstructive pulmonary disease. Am J Respir Crit Care Med 174(5):524–529

Mannino DM (2005) Epidemiology and global impact of chronic obstructive pulmonary disease. Semin Respir Crit Care Med 26(2):204–210

Marino W (1991) Intermittent volume cycled mechanical ventilation via nasal mask in patients with respiratory failure due to COPD. Chest 99:681–684

Marti S, Muñoz X, Rios J et al (2006) Body weight and comorbidity predict mortality in COPD patients treated with oxygen therapy. Eur Respir J 27(4):689–696

McEvoy RD, Pierce RJ, Hillman D et al (2009) Nocturnal non-invasive nasal ventilation in stable hypercapnic COPD: a randomised controlled trial. Thorax 64(7):561–566

McKim DA, Road J, Avendano M et al (2011) Home mechanical ventilation: a Canadian Thoracic Society clinical practice guideline. Can Respir J 18(4):197–215

Meecham Jones DJ, Paul EA, Jones PW, Wedzicha JA (1995) Nasal pressure support ventilation plus oxygen compared with oxygen therapy alone in hypercapnic COPD. Am J Respir Crit Care Med 152(2):538–544

Murray CJL, Lopez AD (1996) The global burden of disease: a comprehensive assessment of mortality and disability from diseases, injuries and risk factors in 1990 and projected to 2020. In: Murray CJL, Lopez AD (eds) Global burden of disease and risk factors. Harvard University Press, Cambridge

Nava S, Fanfulla F, Frigerio P, Navalesi P (2001) Physiologic evaluation of 4 weeks of nocturnal nasal positive pressure ventilation in stable hypercapnic patients with chronic obstructive pulmonary disease. Respiration 68(6):573–583

Nocturnal Oxygen Therapy Trial Group (1980) Continuous or nocturnal oxygen therapy in hypoxemic chronic obstructive lung disease: a clinical trial. Ann Intern Med 93(3):391–398

Osman IM, Godden DJ, Friend JA et al (1997) Quality of life and hospital re-admission in patients with chronic obstructive pulmonary disease. Thorax 52(1):67–71

Rizzi M, Grassi M, Pecis M et al (2009) A specific home care program improves the survival of patients with chronic obstructive pulmonary disease receiving long term oxygen therapy. Arch Phys Med Rehabil 90(3):395–401

Seemungal TA, Donaldson GC, Bhowmik A et al (2000) Time course and recovery of exacerbations in patients with chronic obstructive pulmonary diseases. Am J Respir Crit Care Med 161(5):1608–1613

Seneff MG, Wagner DP, Wagner RP et al (1995) Hospital and 1-year survival of patients admitted to intensive care units with acute exacerbation of chronic obstructive pulmonary disease. JAMA 274(23):1852–1857

Soler-Cataluña JJ, Martìnez-Garcìa MA, Romàn Sànchez P et al (2005) Severe acute exacerbations and mortality in patients with chronic obstructive pulmonary disease. Thorax 60(11):925–931

Strumpf DA, Millman RP, Carlisle CC et al (1991) Nocturnal positive-pressure ventilation via nasal mask in patients with severe chronic obstructive pulmonary disease. Am Rev Respir Dis 144(6):1234–1239

Stuart-Harris Ch et al (1981) Long term domiciliary oxygen therapy in chronic hypoxic cor pulmonale complicating chronic bronchitis and emphysema. The Lancet 1(8222):681–686 (Report of the Medical Research Council Working Party)

Struik FM, Lacasse Y, Goldstein R, Kerstjens HM, Wijkstra PJ (2013) Nocturnal non-invasive positive pressure ventilation for stable chronic obstructive pulmonary disease (Review). Cochrane Database Syst Rev 6:CD002878 doi: 10.1002/14651858.CD002878.pub2.

Teschler H, Stampa J, Ragette R et al (1999) Effect of mouth leak on effectiveness of nasal bilevel ventilatory assistance and sleep architecture. Eur Respir J 14(6):1251–1257

Tuggey JM, Plant PK, Elliot MW (2003) Domiciliary non-invasive ventilation for recurrent acidotic exacerbations of COPD: an economic analysis. Thorax 58(10):867–871

Vestbo J, Hurd SS, Agustí AG, Jones PW, Vogelmeier C, Anzueto A, Barnes PJ, Fabbri LM, Martinez FJ, Nishimura M, Stockley RA, Sin DD, Rodriguez-Roisin R (2013) Global strategy for the diagnosis, management, and prevention of chronic obstructive pulmonary disease: GOLD executive summary. Am J Respir Crit Care Med 187(4):347–365. doi:10.1164/rccm. 201204-0596PP

Wijkstra PJ, Lacasse Y, Guyatt GH et al (2003) A meta-analysis of nocturnal noninvasive positive pressure ventilation in patients with stable COPD. Chest 124(1):337–343

Ventilation in Patients with Restrictive Disorders

22

As we mentioned previously, long-term mechanical ventilation was developed in the 1950s following an epidemic of poliomyelitis. This therapeutic strategy subsequently spread widely and became used in other pathological conditions, including both neuromuscular disorders (particularly myopathies) and restrictive disorders of the chest and lungs (kyphoscoliosis, sequelae of tuberculosis). In recent years the use of this therapeutic strategy has expanded further following the systematic inclusion of patients with amyotrophic lateral sclerosis.

Most of the studies published in the literature are observational or noncontrolled, but their conclusions are in general agreement that mechanical ventilation can improve alveolar ventilation, respiratory function, the strength of respiratory muscles, respiratory drive, and gas exchange as a result of restoring a more physiological ventilation/perfusion ratio. The data obtained in these studies have been confirmed by the few randomized, controlled trials that have been performed, which have shown an improvement in blood gases and sleep quality.

The data available were critically reviewed by the Cochrane Collaboration in 2007, to which we refer you for the analytic details of the studies considered and the statistical methods (Annane et al. 2007). The conclusions of the metaanalysis were unequivocal: the current evidence regarding a therapeutic benefit from mechanical ventilation in restrictive disorders is weak but statistically significant, indicating a reduction in symptoms related to chronic alveolar hypoventilation, at least in the short term. Survival appears to be improved, especially in patients with motor neuron disease. The authors of the metaanalysis concluded by stating that, with the exception of motor neuron disease, further randomized studies are necessary to confirm the beneficial effects in the long term, in particular those regarding quality of life, morbidity, mortality, and cost–benefit ratio and to evaluate the better ventilation technique (i.e., pressure or volume mode).

Except for the last point, it is unlikely that clinicians or ethical committees would accept carrying out a study in this group of patients in whom the accepted clinical practice is recourse to chronic ventilation therapy when they develop signs and symptoms of nocturnal alveolar hypoventilation and/or the presence of hypercapnia during the day. In this regard it is worth reading Hill's editorial,

S. Nava and F. Fanfulla, *Non Invasive Artificial Ventilation*,
DOI: 10.1007/978-88-470-5526-1_22, © Springer-Verlag Italia 2014

"Enough is enough," accompanying a study published by Vianello and colleagues involving a group of patients with Duchenne's muscular dystrophy and chronic respiratory failure (Hill 1994; Vianello et al. 1994). There is, however, room for some critical considerations.

Patients with kyphoscoliosis or sequelae of pulmonary tuberculosis or polio-myelitis are fairly homogeneous and the data in the literature can, therefore be considered consolidated. All the studies carried out in patients with these conditions are concordant in showing improved survival with the use of chronic ventilation therapy, especially intermittent positive pressure ventilation, as shown in various series of French, Dutch, English, and North American patients. Finally, in 2008 a new article was published in Chest reporting the findings of a study carried out in Sweden on a cohort of 188 patients with chronic respiratory failure as a result of sequelae of tuberculosis (Jäger et al. 2008). Of these patients, with a mean age of over 70 years, 103 received LTOT alone, while the other 85 were treated with mechanical ventilation, in most cases in a non invasive manner (15 of these patients also received oxygen therapy). This study essentially represented daily clinical activity, at least in that country, since the data analyzed were collected from the Swedish registry of home oxygen therapy and domiciliary ventilation therapy. As evidence of this, the authors reported a large variability in clinical behavior within the country: in some areas only oxygen therapy was prescribed and in others only mechanical ventilation was used. Nevertheless, the data all pointed in the same direction: there was a difference in mortality between the two groups, with a clear disadvantage for patients receiving only long-term oxygen therapy. After correcting for all confounding factors, the use of NIV was associated with a highly statistically significant marked reduction in mortality risk (risk of death 0.35; confidence interval 0.17–0.7). Similar results were noted by the same authors in a cohort of patients with kyphoscoliosis.

NIV has been demonstrated to improve quality of life and quality of sleep in patients with chronic hypercapnic respiratory failure due to restrictive thoracic disorders. Contal et al. (2011), reviewing the chart of patients who underwent sleep studies before and during NIV for respiratory failure observed reductions in total sleep time (TST), decreased sleep efficiency, overrepresentation of Stage 1 of NREM sleep and reductions in REM sleep, moderate to severe sleep fragmentation because of repeated arousals, and reductions of oxygen saturation with severe desaturations. During NIV they observed great improvement of several sleep parameters: improvement of sleep efficiency and REM sleep with reduction of sleep fragmentation; improvement of nocturnal oxygenation with a mean nocturnal SpO_2 above 90 %, and a decrease in desaturation index.

Unfortunately, the same uniformity of data is difficult to obtain for patients with neuromuscular diseases. The main reason is the diversity of the underlying conditions, which are extremely heterogeneous with regards to both age at onset and evolution. The two neuromuscular disorders mostly extensively studied in this context are undoubtedly Duchenne's muscular dystrophy and amyotrophic lateral sclerosis. The natural history of these conditions, in particular their progression toward chronic respiratory failure, is now better understood and it is, therefore, possible to plan a personalized follow-up protocol for each patient.

22.1 Duchenne's Muscular Dystrophy

As just mentioned, the natural history of Duchenne's muscular dystrophy is well-known, being characterized by a progressive loss of lung volume following total loss of ambulation and consequent confinement to a wheelchair; when the vital capacity falls below 1 L, the 5-year survival rate is 8 %. Episodes of nocturnal desaturation usually appear after this stage, with the development of global respiratory failure at the age of about 18–20 years. The onset of daytime hypercapnia is a very important marker of clinical severity since the life expectancy of patients with this sign is 9–10 months on average. The systematic use of ventilation therapy in patients with Duchenne's muscular dystrophy has raised the mean age of death in these patients from 19 to 25 years, with 1- and 5-year survival rates of 85 % and 73 %, respectively.

The history of chronic ventilation treatment in Duchenne's muscular dystrophy has had its ups and downs, especially after the publication in 1994 of a French study demonstrating a worsening of prognosis in patients undergoing ventilation therapy (Raphael et al. 1994). This study was performed to test the hypothesis that early use of nocturnal ventilation therapy could play a role in delaying the deterioration in respiratory function, in particular the onset of respiratory failure. Seventy patients with a documented initial decline in vital capacity were enrolled into the study. The method of enrollment and the treatment modalities were heavily criticized (a posteriori). Most of the criticisms regarded the absence of a specific cardiological evaluation, the fact that humidifiers were not used, and the lack of data on respiratory function during sleep. In fact, an a posteriori analysis limited to 19 patients (10 of whom in the experimental group) who had symptoms of nocturnal hypoventilation showed that NIV caused an improvement in blood gases in the short term and in the longer term (1 year) provided some relief from the symptoms associated with nocturnal hypoventilation.

The American guidelines, proposed by the American Thoracic Society, recommend the use of NIV in patients with obstructive sleep apnea (OSA), a phenomenon particularly common in these patients, or in the presence of chronic respiratory failure (American Thoracic Society 2004). In fact, in 1994 Vianello and colleagues found in a controlled, but not randomized, study that five patients with advanced stage Duchenne's muscular dystrophy treated with NIV were still alive after 2 years, whereas four out the five patients who had refused this treatment had died (Vianello et al. 1994). The identification of the best time to start ventilation treatment in this group of patients has always been a crucial issue. Ward and colleagues carried out a randomized, controlled trial in a group of patients with neuromuscular disorders, including Duchenne's muscular dystrophy, who had documented nocturnal alveolar hypoventilation but normal daytime levels of blood CO_2. The patients were divided into two groups: one group received ventilation therapy during the night, while the other formed the control group. In this second group, NIV could be commenced in those patients who, during the 2-year follow-up, developed daytime hypercapnia, more than three episodes of bronchopulmonary infection or uncontrollable symptoms of alveolar hypoventilation. The results were unequivocal: 70 % of patients in the control group had to start ventilation therapy already within the first year of the follow-up; by the end of the second year, 90 % of the patients in the control group were receiving chronic ventilation treatment (Ward et al. 2005).

22.2   Indications for NIV in Patients with Restrictive Chest Diseases or with Restrictive Chest Diseases

The most recent guidelines or position statements suggest starting NIV in patients with daytime symptoms of hypoventilation and hypercapnia or nocturnal desaturations (SpO_2 < 88 % for more than 5 min consecutively). In the more progressive neuromuscular disorders NIV is recommended if symptoms of nocturnal hypoventilation or orthopnea are present in patients with a maximum inspiratory pressure (MIP) at the mouth of <60 % of predicted or a vital capacity <50 % of predicted. Table 22.1 summarizes the indications for home ventilation therapy in patients with restrictive chest diseases and/or neuromuscular disorders. Intermittent negative pressure ventilation was gradually abandoned with the advent of positive pressure ventilators (volume or pressure support) specifically studied for use at home. The decisions on the mode of ventilation and the type of mask to use are essentially left to the choice/preference of the doctor and patient. Surprisingly, there are no data available in the literature on a systematic comparison of the different methods of positive pressure ventilation in this type of patient. The daily reality, as determined from a survey in Europe, indicates that the use of pressure support prevails over volume support. However, we believe that this aspect should

Table 22.1 Indications for starting NIV

Indications for ventilation therapy	
Absolute	Daytime $PaCO_2$ >45 mmHg
Or	Orthopnea or symptoms of nocturnal hypoventilation (morning headache, daytime sleepiness, disturbed sleep with frequent awakenings)
In association with one of the following:	• Vital capacity <50 % of theoretical[a]
	• MIP/MEP < 60 % theoretical
	• Nocturnal SaO_2 < 88 % for >5 min consecutively
	• Frequent exacerbations

[a]This cut-off may differ according to the underlying disease

be investigated more thoroughly in the future, particularly in those patients who are moving toward progressive ventilator dependence. Table 22.2 presents the possible advantages and disadvantages of the two types of ventilation.

As far as concerns the ventilation masks, a study carried out in a group of patients with chronic respiratory failure showed that nasal masks are better tolerated than oronasal masks or systems using nasal pillows. The oronasal masks do, however, seem to be more effective in lowering the level of CO_2.

These data are in line with clinical experience, which seems to favor the use of nasal masks as the reference interface for long-term NIV. In any case, patients with excessive air loss through the mouth or with advanced bulbar involvement could be better managed with oronasal interfaces. These masks should have a safety valve and a quick release system to minimize the risks of asphyxia, if the ventilator fails or aspiration, in the case of vomiting. The use of ventilation via the mouth (usually during the daytime) plays an important role in long-term ventilation treatment of patients with neuromuscular disease who are heavily dependent on the respirator: together with nocturnal nasal ventilation this enables long-term, even continuous, NIV with a good level of comfort and a low risk of developing pressure sores.

Table 22.2 Main differences between intermittent positive pressure volume and pressure support ventilators

Volume support ventilators	
Advantages	Stable tidal volume
	Silent
	Less energy consumption, so batteries last longer
	Can be used during maneuvers to help coughing
	Oral ventilation
Disadvantages	Often heavy
	Management of the alarms
Pressure support ventilators	
Advantages	Light
	Less expensive
	Compensation for air leaks from the mask
	Alarms can be deactivated
Disadvantages	Noisier
	EPAP always present
	Tidal volume not always guaranteed
	Cannot be used during maneuvers to help coughing
	Oral ventilation difficult

Suggested Reading

Annane D, Orlikowski D, Chevret S et al (2007) Nocturnal mechanical ventilation for chronic hypoventilation in patients with neuromuscular and chest wall disorders. Cochrane Database Syst Rev 4:CD001941

Ambrosino N, Carpenè N, Gherardi M (2009) Chronic respiratory care for neuromuscular diseases in adults. Eur Respir J 34:444–451

Bach JR, Alba AS, Saporito LR (1993) Intermittent positive pressure ventilation via the mouth as an alternative to tracheostomy for 257 ventilator users. Chest 103(1):174–182

Bach JR, Robert D, Leger P, Langevin B (1995) Sleep fragmentation in kyphoscoliotic individuals with alveolar hypoventilation treated with NIPPV. Chest 107(6):1552–1558

Bach JR, Rajaraman R, Ballanger F et al (1998) Neuromuscular ventilatory insufficiency: effect of home mechanical ventilator use vs oxygen therapy on pneumonia and hospitalization rates. Am J Phys Med Rehabil 77(1):8–19

Barbé F, Quera-Salva MA, de Lattre J et al (1996) Long-term effects of nasal intermittent positive pressure ventilation on pulmonary function and sleep architecture in patients with neuromuscular diseases. Chest 110(5):1179–1183

Baydur A, Layne E, Aral H et al (2000) Long term non-invasive ventilation in the community for patients with musculoskeletal disorders: 46 years experience and review. Thorax 55(1):4–11

Bersanini C, Khirani S, Ramirez A et al (2012) Nocturnal hypoxaemia and hypercapnia in children with neuromuscular disorders. Eur Respir J 39:1206–1212

Bourke SC, Tomlinson M, Williams TL et al (2006) Effects of non-invasive ventilation on survival and quality of life in patients with amyotrophic lateral sclerosis: a randomised controlled trial. Lancet Neurol 5(2):140–147

Bushby K, Finkel R, Birnkrant DJ et al (2010) Diagnosis and management of duchenne muscular dystrophy, part 2: implementation of multidisciplinary care. Lancet Neurol 9:177–189

Cazzolli PA, Oppenheimer EA (1996) Home mechanical ventilation for amyotrophic lateral sclerosis: nasal compared to tracheostomy-intermittent positive pressure ventilation. J Neurol Sci 139(Suppl):123–128

Contal O, Janssens JP, Dury M, Delguste P, Aubert G, Rodenstein D (2011) Sleep in ventilator failure in restrictive thoracic disorders. effects of treatment with non invasive ventilation. Sleep Med 12:373–377

Duiverman ML, Bladder G, Meinesz AF, Wijkstra PJ (2006) Home mechanical ventilatory support in patients with restrictive ventilatory disorders: a 48-year experience. Respir Med 100(1):56–65

Ellis ER, Bye PT, Bruderer JW, Sullivan CE (1987) Treatment of respiratory failure during sleep in patients with neuromuscular disease. Positive-pressure ventilation through a nose mask. Am Rev Respir Dis 135(1):148–152

Finder JD, Birnkrant D, Carl J et al [American Thoracic Society] (2004) Respiratory care of the patient with Duchenne muscular dystrophy: ATS consensus statement. Am J Respir Crit Care Med 170(4):456-465

Gonzalez J, Sharshar T, Hart N et al (2003) Air leaks during mechanical ventilation as a cause of persistent hypercapnia in neuromuscular disorders. Intensive Care Med 29(4):596–602

Gustafson T, Franklin KA, Midgren B et al (2006) Survival of patients with kyphoscoliosis receiving mechanical ventilation or oxygen at home. Chest 130(6):1828–1833

Hill NS (1994) Noninvasive positive pressure ventilation in neuromuscular disease. Enough is enough! Chest 105(2):337–338

Hull J, Aniapravan R, Chan E et al (2012). British Thoracic Society guideline for respiratory management of children with neuromuscular weakness. Thorax 67:i1ei40. doi: 10.1136/thoraxjnl-2012-201964

Jäger L, Franklin KA, Midgren B et al (2008) Increased survival with mechanical ventilation in posttuberculosis patients with the combination of respiratory failure and chest wall deformity. Chest 133(1):156–160

Lechtzin N, Scott Y, Busse AM et al (2007) Early use of non-invasive ventilation prolongs survival in subjects with ALS. Amyotroph Lateral Scler 8:185–188

Leger P, Bedicam JM, Cornette A et al (1994) Nasal intermittent positive pressure ventilation. Longterm follow-up in patients with severe chronic respiratory insufficiency. Chest 105(1):100–105

Masa JF, Celli BR, Riesco JA et al (1997) Noninvasive positive pressure ventilation and not oxygen may prevent overt ventilatory failure in patients with chest wall diseases. Chest 112(1):207–213

Navalesi P, Fanfulla F, Frigerio P et al (2000) Physiologic evaluation of noninvasive mechanical ventilation delivered with three types of masks in patients with chronic hypercapnic respiratory failure. Crit Care Med 28(6):1785–1790

Oppenheimer EA (1995) Amyotrophic lateral sclerosis: care, survival and quality of life on homemechanical ventilation. In: Robert D, Make BJ, Leger P et al (eds) Home mechanical ventilation. Arnette Blackwell, Paris

Pinto AC, Evangelista T, Carvalho M et al (1995) Respiratory assistance with a non-invasive ventilator (Bipap) in MND/ALS patients: survival rates in a controlled trial. J Neurol Sci 129(Suppl):19–26

Piper AJ, Sullivan CE (1996) Effects of long-term nocturnal nasal ventilation on spontaneous breathing during sleep in neuromuscular and chest wall disorders. Eur Respir J 9(7):1515–1522

Raphael JC, Chevret S, Chastang C, Bouvet F (1994) Randomised trial of preventive nasal ventilation in Duchenne muscular dystrophy. French multicentre cooperative study group on home mechanical assistance in Duchenne de Boulogne muscular dystrophy. Lancet 343(8913):1600–1604

Restrick LJ, Fox NC, Braid G et al (1993) Comparison of nasal pressure support ventilation with nasal intermittent positive pressure ventilation in patients with nocturnal hypoventilation. Eur Respir J 6(3):364–370

Robert D, Gérard M, Leger P et al (1983) [Permanent mechanical ventilation at home via a tracheostomy in chronic respiratory insufficiency]. La ventilation mechanique a domicile definitive par tracheostomie de l'insuffisant respiratoire chronique. Rev Fr Mal Respir 11(6):923–936

Schönhofer B (2002) Choice of ventilator types, modes, and settings for long-term ventilation. Respir Care Clin N Am 8(3):419–445

Simonds AK, Elliott MW (1995) Outcome of domiciliary nasal intermittent positive pressure ventilation in restrictive and obstructive disorders. Thorax 50(6):604–609

Simonds AK (2006) Recent advances in respiratory care for neuromuscular disease. Chest 130(6):1879–1886

Teschler H, Stampa J, Ragette R et al (1999) Effect of mouth leak on effectiveness of nasal bilevel ventilatory assistance and sleep architecture. Eur Respir J 14(6):1251–1257

Vianello A, Bevilacqua M, Salvador V et al (1994) Long-term nasal intermittent positive pressure ventilation in advanced Duchenne's muscular dystrophy. Chest 105(2):445–448

Ward S, Chatwin M, Heather S, Simonds AK (2005) Randomised controlled trial of non-invasive ventilation (NIV) for nocturnal hypoventilation in neuromuscular and chest wall disease patients with daytime normocapnia. Thorax 60(12):1019–1024

Willson GN, Piper AJ, Norman M et al (2004) Nasal versus full face mask for noninvasive ventilation in chronic respiratory failure. Eur Respir J 23(4):605–609

Rationale for Ventilation Therapy During Sleep

23

23.1 Physiology

Sleep is normally associated with significant changes in many physiological functions, including respiration. The most important differences between wakefulness and sleep are body position, control of breathing, changes in resistance to flow, the ventilatory response to changes in work load, and the coordinated activation of the respiratory muscles.

During sleep there is an approximately 10–15 % reduction in the minute volume, essentially caused by a decrease in the tidal volume without appreciable modifications in the respiratory rate. These changes are primarily due to a decrease in metabolic requirements, a marked increase in upper airway resistance, and a reduced ventilatory response to the increased load. Arterial blood gases settle around values that are obviously different from those during wakefulness, with a reduction of approximately 4–10 mmHg in the PaO_2 and an increase of about 3–7 mmHg in the $PaCO_2$. The ventilatory response to changes in blood gases is different, usually being less during sleep than while awake. For example, the set point of CO_2, that is, the value of the partial pressure of CO_2 in the blood at which ventilation starts to increase, is higher during sleep than while awake and the slope of the linear relationship between the level of ventilation and the blood CO_2 appears to be reduced, both when breathing room air and in conditions of hyperoxia or hypoxia.

The magnitude of these changes is related to the stages of deep sleep with maximum stability of the control systems. In fact, during the transition phases between sleep and wakefulness, breathing can be irregular with episodes of central apnea and clusters of periodic breathing. Obviously, there is large inter-individual variability in all the aspects considered so far. In fact, Dunroy and colleagues analyzed a group of normal subjects while awake and during sleep, measuring changes in the partial pressure of CO_2 at end expiration ($PETCO_2$) in normal conditions and when breathing through a dead space, correlating these changes with the level of ventilatory response to the hypercapnic stimulus. In awake patients no significant relationship was seen between the changes in the $PETCO_2$ and the slope of the

S. Nava and F. Fanfulla, *Non Invasive Artificial Ventilation*,
DOI: 10.1007/978-88-470-5526-1_23, © Springer-Verlag Italia 2014

response to hypercapnia; in contrast, during sleep the individuals with a lower ventilatory response to hypercapnia had a greater increase of $PETCO_2$ (up to 8 mmHg) during application of the dead space (Dunroy et al. 2003).

The changes in blood gases are not only due to physiological variations in the level of ventilation. In fact, the functional residual capacity is smaller during sleep than during wakefulness: the reduction is 7 % during non-rapid eye movement (NREM) sleep and more during rapid eye movement (REM) sleep. There are various reasons for this decrease in functional residual capacity: central pooling of blood, a decrease in lung compliance, reduced tone of the respiratory muscles, and early closure of the peripheral airways. The physiological changes in the distribution of ventilation and lung aeration during sleep were studied by Appelberg and colleagues, who used a new spiral computed tomography method in a group of ten healthy subjects (Appelberg et al. 2007). While the subjects were awake, there were no significant changes in the gas/tissue ratio, functional residual capacity, or cranial-caudal distribution of aeration, while an increase in lung density was confirmed passing from the ventral regions to the dorsal ones. In contrast, during sleep the authors found a 9 % reduction in aeration of the dorsal regions compared to the aeration during wakefulness and an opposite trend in the ventral regions with an increase of 6 %. The reduction in aeration observed in the dorsal regions of the lung during sleep was correlated significantly with the functional residual capacity recorded while the subjects were awake: the greater the functional residual capacity, the less the reduction in lung volume while asleep. These data confirm that a reduction in muscle tone and the decrease in functional residual capacity with closure of the dependent small airways are the major factors causing the loss of lung volume observed during sleep.

The activity of the respiratory muscles also undergoes substantial changes during sleep. The first change is a decrease in the tonic activity of the dilating muscles of the upper airways, which causes a marked increase in the resistance of the upper airways. The activity of the pump muscle is obviously not modified significantly during the NREM phases of sleep. The situation changes radically during REM sleep: in this phase the whole respiratory activity is sustained by the diaphragm because of the lack of tone of the antigravity muscles. Indeed, there are data suggesting an increase in the electrical activity of the diaphragm during the REM phase of sleep, although the effect is lost because of a loss of efficiency in the neuro-mechanical coupling observed during this particular phase of sleep. In fact, during ocular movements, the so-called phasic REM sleep, there is considerable irregularity in the electrical activity of the diaphragm with the appearance or increase of paradoxical respiration, brief episodes of central apnea and further irregularity of the respiratory pattern (Fig. 23.1).

In conclusion, important physiological changes in respiratory activity occur during sleep. These changes are mainly under chemical control and the control systems continue to work although the thresholds of "intervention" are obviously higher. In other words, the body reacts regularly only in the presence of major changes (for example, large variations in blood gases, mechanical load supported, etc.) and in the only way possible, that is, by waking, which restores the typical

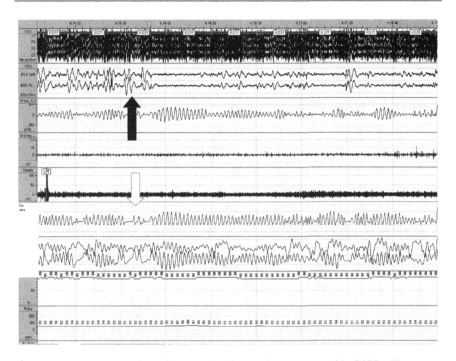

Fig. 23.1 Four-minute period of REM sleep in an obese patient with COPD. The arrows indicate eye movements and the presence of paradoxical respiration (see the text for more detailed information)

conditions of the state of being awake. This delicate balance between needing to maintain sleep as constant as possible and ensuring correct homeostasis is obviously subject to great individual variability, not only in the respiratory variables considered above, but also in those related to the sleep itself (type, arousability, age-dependent differences, etc.).

23.2 Pathological Conditions

Sleep is a crucial period for respiration, for the reasons set out previously. Respiratory abnormalities during sleep are currently a group of disorders that are of great interest both epidemiologically and from the point of view of healthcare management.

From a nosographic point of view we describe disorders that occur exclusively during sleep and preexisting pathological conditions which take on particular characteristics during sleep (Table 23.1). In this chapter we will deal essentially with the pathophysiological mechanisms that cause hypoxemia and hypercapnia during sleep.

Table 23.1 The clinical pictures of the most common respiratory alterations during sleep

Respiratory disorders present exclusively during sleep	Respiratory disorders with characteristic signs during sleep	Non-respiratory disorders with respiratory alterations during sleep
OSAS	COPD	Chronic heart failure
Central apnea syndrome	Nocturnal asthma	Neurological disorders (e.g., stroke, Parkinson disease)
Obesity-hypoventilation syndrome	Diaphragmatic disorders/chest cage deformities	Neuromuscular disorders
	Idiopathic alveolar hypoventilation	

The current definition (Table 23.2) of nocturnal desaturation/hypoxemia secondary to a preexisting pathology requires:

- at least 30 % of the total sleep time spent with oxyhemoglobin saturation <90 % (definition proposed by the French school of authors) or, alternatively, at least 5 min of sleep with an oxyhemoglobin saturation <90 % and a nadir value <85 %, with the majority of this time occurring during the REM phase of sleep (definition proposed by the North-American school of authors);
- the absence of other conditions that could explain these changes (other disorders, use/abuse of pharmacological agents or substances, etc.).
  The proposed definitions of alveolar hypoventilation during sleep are:
- an increase of at least 10 mmHg in the $PaCO_2$ during sleep compared to the level observed in the supine position in the period awake prior to sleeping [standard proposed by the American Academy of Sleep Medicine (AASM)];
- nocturnal blood-gas analysis showing hypercapnia or an increase in $PaCO_2$ not proportional to that observed during wakefulness [according to the International Classification of Diseases (ICD) IX].

The main pathophysiological mechanisms causing changes in ventilation during sleep are summarised in Table 23.3, while Table 23.4 lists the principle clinical symptoms of nocturnal alveolar hypoventilation. In general, patients with multiple chronic conditions can have lower values of partial pressure of oxygen (PaO_2) during sleep than those found while they are awake. Changes in gas exchange during sleep and their prognostic impact have been particularly thoroughly studied in patients with COPD, a pathological condition that we will deal with extensively, not only because of its obvious epidemiological relevance, but also because nocturnal home oxygen therapy was proposed initially and exclusively for this disorder. A state of hypoxemia while awake tends to worsen during sleep, but the depth of the nocturnal desaturation can differ markedly between patients, independently of the PaO_2 values while awake.

Table 23.2 Diagnostic criteria for sleep-related hypoventilation/hypoxemia syndromes

Disorder	Diagnostic criteria
Sleep-related idiopathic alveolar hypoventilation	A. Polysomnography shows episodes of fast, shallow breathing for more than 10 s associated with desaturations and frequent arousals associated with respiratory alterations or brady-tachycardia
	B. Absence of primary lung disorders, skeletal deformities or peripheral neuromuscular disorders that could affect ventilation
	C. The condition cannot be better explained by various other types of disorders (sleep, internal, neurological, mental, use/abuse of substances or pharmacological agents)
Congenital alveolar hypoventilation	A. In the perinatal period the patient has shallow breathing, or cyanosis with apnea, during sleep
	B. The hypoventilation is worse during sleep than when awake
	C. The ventilatory response to hypoxia or hypercapnia is absent or decreased
	D. Polysomnography shows severe hypoxia with hypercapnia, generally without apnea
	E. The condition cannot be better explained by various other types of sleep disorder, other medical or neurological factors, use/abuse of substances or pharmacological agents
Sleep-related hypoxemia/hypoventilation due to abnormalities of lung parenchyma or vascular conditions	A. Presence of parenchymal lung disorders or vascular conditions considered to be the main cause of the hypoxemia
	B. Polysomnography or arterial blood-gas analyses carried out during sleep show at least one of the following signs:
	• An SaO_2 during sleep < 90 % for at least 5 min with a nadir ≤ 85 %
	• At least 30 % of the total sleep time with $SaO_2 < 90$ %
	• Blood-gases during sleep: very high $PaCO_2$ or a disproportionate increase with respect to values recorded while awake
	C. The condition cannot be better explained by other sleep disorders, other medical or neurological factors, use/abuse of substances or pharmacological agents

(continued)

Table 23.2 (continued)

Disorder	Diagnostic criteria
Sleep-related hypoxemia/hypoventilation due to chronic obstruction of the lower airways	A. Presence of chronic bronchial obstruction (FEV_1 < 70 % of predicted) considered to be the main cause of the hypoxemia
	B. Polysomnography or arterial blood-gas analyses carried out during sleep show at least one of the following signs:
	• An SaO_2 during sleep < 90 % for at least 5 min with a nadir ≤ 85 %
	• At least 30 % of the total sleep time with SaO_2 < 90 %
	• Blood-gases during sleep: very high $PaCO_2$ or a disproportionate increase with respect to values recorded while awake
	C. The condition cannot be better explained by other sleep disorders, other medical or neurological factors, use/abuse of substances or pharmacological agents
Sleep-related hypoxemia/hypoventilation due to neuromuscular or chest cage disorders	A. A neuromuscular or chest wall disorder considered to be the main cause of the hypoxemia
	B. Polysomnography or arterial blood-gas analyses carried out during sleep show at least one of the following signs:
	• An SaO_2 during sleep < 90 % for at least 5 min with a nadir ≤ 85 %
	• At least 30 % of the total sleep time with SaO_2 < 90 %
	• Blood-gases during sleep: very high $PaCO_2$ or a disproportionate increase with respect to values recorded while awake
	C. The condition cannot be better explained by other sleep disorders, other medical or neurological factors, use/abuse of substances or pharmacological agents

The results of lung function tests correlate poorly with the degree of nocturnal hypoxemia, because this is affected by any comorbidities present, such as heart failure and obstructive apnea during sleep. Desaturations during sleep occur more frequently in the REM phase, both in patients with COPD and in those with other disorders, but may also be observed during the NREM phase, in particular in stages I and II of sleep, when they are usually less deep and shorter lasting. There is, however, often a relationship between the values of PaO_2 while awake and

Table 23.3 Main risk factors for the onset of respiratory disorders during sleep and their related mechanisms

Risk factors	Mechanisms
Hypoventilation during REM phase sleep	Atony of antigravity muscles. The diaphragm is the only muscle that sustains ventilation
Weakness of the diaphragm	Can be isolated or part of widespread muscular alterations. Maximum impairment while lying supine in REM phase sleep
Increased resistance of the upper airways	Weakness of the bulbar muscles. Hypotonicity of muscles that dilate the pharynx during REM phase sleep. Anatomical changes (retrognathia, macroglossia). Adenotonsillar hypertrophy, recurrent infections of the upper airways, atopic state (all frequent conditions in growing children)
Restrictive ventilation syndrome	Deformities of the chest cage. Scoliosis. Obesity. Pulmonary atelectasia with the onset of nocturnal desaturations
Reduced chemoreceptor sensitivity	Chronic sleep deprivation. Chronic hypoventilation with increased serum bicarbonate. Primary abnormality of the respiratory centers or carotid body
Alterations to the central nervous system	Primary hypersomnia

Table 23.4 Main symptoms associated with nocturnal alveolar hypoventilation

Signs and symptoms often associated with nocturnal alveolar hypoventilation
Onset of dyspnea during common daily life activities
Orthopnea in patients with changes to the diaphragm
Poor sleep quality: insomnia, nightmares, frequent awakenings
Headache during the night or when wakening
Daytime symptoms such as sleepiness, fatigue, asthenia, loss of strength
Worsening of intellectual performance
Loss of appetite and weight loss
Recurrent complications (respiratory infections)
Clinical signs of cor pulmonale

those during sleep: in fact, subjects with lower PaO_2 values while awake have a more severe picture while asleep. This correlation is mainly due to the shape of the dissociation curve of hemoglobin: the same reduction in amplitude of the value of PaO_2 has different consequences depending on the starting value of SaO_2. The amplitude of the desaturations is greater when the starting value of SaO_2 is close to or less than 90 %.

Many of the functional variables studied differ between patients with COPD who have episodes of nocturnal desaturation and those who do not have desaturations. Toraldo and colleagues showed that the functional indices best identifying patients with nocturnal desaturation are the percentage of time spent with $SaO_2 < 90\%$ (T90), mean pulmonary artery pressure, and values of $PaCO_2$ (Toraldo et al. 2005).

The role played by nocturnal desaturations in the natural history of COPD has not yet been completely clarified. Researchers have concentrated most attention on patients with PaO_2 values > 60 mmHg, that is, with modest or no daytime hypoxemia. It has been proposed that the nocturnal desaturations occurring in subjects without significant daytime hypoxemia could induce the development of permanent pulmonary hypertension, accelerating the onset of cor pulmonale. Fletcher and colleagues demonstrated that patients who desaturated during the night had a lower survival rate compared to those who did not have nocturnal desaturations (Fletcher et al. 1991). One of their subsequent studies seemed to suggest that patients whose episodes of nocturnal desaturation were treated with oxygen therapy had a better survival than patients who did not receive this treatment (Fletcher et al. 1992). The difference between the two groups was, however, at the limit of statistical significance. Subsequently Chaouat and colleagues did not find that patients with nocturnal desaturations had higher pulmonary artery pressures than patients who did not have desaturations (1997). Two other studies on the survival of patients with COPD receiving long-term oxygen therapy for moderate hypoxemia (Gòrecka and Veale) yielded similar results: long-term oxygen therapy does not improve survival in this type of patient. Finally, Chaouat and colleagues (2001), in a follow-up study lasting 2 years, showed that the presence of isolated nocturnal hypoxemia, or worsening of moderate hypoxemia during sleep, does not promote the development of pulmonary arterial hypertension or cause a worsening of daytime gases.

However, in a prospective study with a follow-up of 42 months, Sergi and colleagues demonstrated that desaturations could be an independent risk factor for the development of chronic respiratory failure in patients with COPD with a daytime $PaO_2 > 60$ mmHg. Finally, other longitudinal studies demonstrated that nocturnal desaturations were more frequent in those patients with a faster decline in pulmonary mechanics, as demonstrated by a more rapid worsening of FEV_1 or by a greater increase in the $PaCO_2$.

The onset of nocturnal desaturations in patients with COPD has been related to various factors, including changes in respiratory mechanics, worsening V/Q mismatch, increased resistance in the airways, and decreased strength of the respiratory muscles. Ballard and colleagues observed that the REM phase of sleep causes a significant reduction in the minute volume related to a decrease in the tidal volume and a marked reduction in neuromuscular drive (Ballard et al. 1995). In contrast, no change was seen in lung volumes or resistance of the lower airways among the states of wakefulness, NREM sleep, and REM sleep. Furthermore, the physiological increase in the resistance in the upper airways during sleep could contribute to the decrease in minute volume. In a subsequent study carried out by Becker and colleagues on a group of patients with various different types of chronic respiratory disease, it was found that the main cause of nocturnal desaturations was the reduction in alveolar ventilation, which was particularly evident during the REM phase of sleep. On the basis of these results, the authors concluded that any treatment to correct desaturation during REM sleep must enable recovery of adequate alveolar ventilation during sleep (Becker et al. 1999).

Patients with COPD have a high workload already during wakefulness because of the chronic obstruction of the airways and a state of alveolar hyperinflation, while patients with restrictive chest disorders mainly have an increased elastic load because of the reduced lung and chest compliance (a state that is very frequent in many neuromuscular disorders). The capacity of the respiratory muscles to generate force in patients with COPD appears to be reduced because of structural and functional abnormalities, and is sometimes so substantial as to prevent an increase in respiratory work. The diaphragm, like other skeletal muscles, responds to an overload with cellular and functional adaptations. However, unlike other skeletal muscles which, after a period of overload, can rest and recover, the activity of the diaphragm cannot be interrupted, producing a state of chronic overload. Furthermore, its capacity to adapt to these unfavorable conditions can be compromised by various factors such as poor nutritional status, prolonged corticosteroid treatment, and chronic hypoxia. Consequently, dysfunction of or damage to the diaphragm can be due to both an excessive resistive load and to adverse clinical factors that challenge and overcome the muscle's capacity for adaptation. Indeed, Macgowan and colleagues showed that the extent of the structural changes to the diaphragm is proportional to the impairment of airflow: the percentage of the area of damaged diaphragm was between 4 and 34 % of the total (Macgowan et al. 2001). In subjects with a less efficient or weak diaphragm, the physiological reduction of the activity of the intercostal and accessory muscles during the REM phase of sleep, as for all the antigravity muscles, causes a significant reduction in inspiratory pressure, thus contributing to the development of alveolar hypoventilation. In patients with advanced COPD or neuromuscular disorders, the inspiratory accessory muscles, such as the sternocleidomastoid muscles, the scalenes and the abdominal muscles, play an important role in increasing ventilation during wakefulness and NREM sleep, but not during REM sleep.

Sleep, particularly the REM phase, is characterized by an increase in the resistance in the upper airways. O'Donoghue and colleagues, studying a group of patients with severe COPD with daytime hypercapnia, observed that the onset of alveolar hypoventilation during sleep was correlated with the level of CO_2 in the blood during wakefulness, the body mass index (BMI), the severity of the limitation in inspiratory flow during REM sleep, and with the apnea/hypopnea index. Consequently, obesity and the reduction of caliber of the upper airways, even in the absence of episodes of apnea or hypopnea, cause a further increase in inspiratory work (O'Donoghue et al. 2003).

At the same time, the authors observed that when the resistive load of the upper airways was decreased during sleep, for example by using a mixture of helium and oxygen, the patients with hypercapnic COPD while awake did not increase their level of ventilation but simply reduced the inspiratory work of the muscles proportionally. This finding confirms that the minute volume is physiologically decreased during sleep in comparison with the usual values during peaceful wakefulness.

However, many patients have more than one sleep-related pathological condition. The association between COPD and obstructive sleep apnea (OSA) was described in the middle of the 1980s by Flenley, who called it "overlap syndrome" (Flenley 1985). Various studies, carried out mainly in selected cohorts of patients, found a high prevalence of OSA in patients with COPD or, conversely, a high prevalence of COPD in patients with OSA. However, the data from the Sleep Heart Health Study did not confirm an increase in the prevalence of OSA in patients with COPD, indicating a simple casual concomitance of two very frequent disorders in the general population and not a pathophysiological connection.

Nevertheless, it was demonstrated that the overlap syndrome predisposes to the development of daytime hypercapnia and hypoxemia, independently of lung function. OSA seems to be an important cause of hypoxemia and hypercapnia in those patients in whom the severity of the changes in gas exchange appears excessive with respect to the degree of deterioration in lung function. Chan and colleagues observed that COPD patients with hypercapnia had a higher number of respiratory disorders during sleep, a higher BMI, and smaller diameter of the upper airways compared to normocapnic patients with a similar picture of respiratory function (Chan et al. 1990).

One important factor to consider, both in the genesis of altered gas exchange during sleep and in the consequences, is the quality of sleep in patients with chronic respiratory disorders. For example, patients with COPD have higher incidences of insomnia, excessive daytime sleepiness, and nightmares compared to the general population. Polysomnographic data show less efficient sleep, a decrease in the REM phase, and numerous transitions between the various stages of sleep. Poor sleep quality could be a factor predisposing to the development of chronic fatigue and the reduced quality of life usually reported by these patients. The mechanisms underlying the changes in sleep structure are under debate and could be related to gas exchange, the assumption of drugs, or the generally compromised state of the patient. Optimization of pharmacological treatment, with improvement in dyspnea also promotes better control of the insomnia. Hypoxia stimulates the reticular activating system and there is a strong association between hypoxemia and number of awakenings or 'micro-awakenings.' However, their frequency does not seem to decrease after nocturnal oxygen therapy, suggesting that it is not the hypoxemia, but rather some related phenomena, such as hypercapnia, that trigger the development of arousals.

Recently, two different follow-up studies clearly demonstrated that the presence of untreated OSA in COPD patients is associated with a very substantial increase in mortality. The first, performed in Spain, involved three groups of relatively young COPD patients (mean age 57 years): patients with overlap syndrome treated with CPAP, patients with overlap syndrome not treated with CPAP, and patients with COPD without OSA. The distribution of COPD severity was similar in the three groups: 80 % of the patients were on stage II or III of GOLD classification of the COPD severity (Marin et al. 2010).

The Authors found that the overlap syndrome was associated with an increased risks of death and hospitalization because of exacerbation of COPD. CPAP treatment was associated with improved survival and decreased hospitalizations in these patients.

The second study, performed in Brazil, involved two groups of patients with severe COPD already in chronic respiratory failure requiring long-term oxygen therapy, who were diagnosed with moderate-to-severe OSAS: one group accepted and were adherent to CPAP treatment, while the second group did not accept or were not adherent and were considered not treated (Machado et al. 2010).

The 5-year survival estimate was 71 and 26 % in the CPAP-treated and non-treated groups, respectively ($p<0.01$). Patients treated with CPAP had a significantly lower risk of death: hazard ratio of death versus non-treated 0.19 (0.08–0.48). The Authors concluded that CPAP treatment was associated with higher survival in patients with moderate-to-severe OSAS and hypoxemic COPD receiving LTOT.

23.3 Chronic Respiratory Failure

Sleep alterations in patients with respiratory failure have not been extensively investigated. Most studies have been performed in acute settings, usually during intensive care with the aim of assessing the impact of the intensive care unit environment on sleep quality (Boyko et al. 2012). These studies generally concluded that sleep quality is altered in patients admitted to ICU for respiratory failure as a result of severity of the illness, environmental noise, light intensity, types and modes of mechanical ventilation, drugs, or care procedures. Different patterns of alterations were observed in these patients: reduction in total amount of sleep, increased light sleep, severe sleep fragmentation, large amount of slow-wave sleep, and a monophasic pattern with continuous low-voltage theta-delta activity. The variability of these pictures is related to the pathophysiology or severity of respiratory failure, clinical status (acute, recovery from acute episode, chronic), and the presence of acidemia, or alkalosis.

23.4 Obstructive Sleep Apnea Syndrome: Obesity-Hypoventilation Syndrome

Obstructive sleep apnea syndrome (OSAS) is a very common pathological condition that is currently considered a real respiratory emergency. The most recent investigations indicate that the prevalence of OSAS (presence of pathological respiratory events associated with symptoms) is approximately 5 % in adult men and 3 % in adult women; however, the difference between the two sexes tends to decrease after the menopause. Considering the presence of respiratory disorders during sleep, independently of whether the patient has symptoms, the prevalence increases greatly, up to 24 %.

OSAS is characterized by recurrent episodes of total or partial obstruction of the upper airways (apnea or hypopnea/inspiratory flow limitation, respectively) which lead to frequent awakenings, episodes of oxyhemoglobin desaturation, oscillations in heart rate, and systemic and pulmonary blood pressures. A variety of studies have clearly defined the impact of this syndrome on mortality, respiratory and cardio-cerebrovascular morbidity, capacity to drive, neuropsychological factors, socioeconomic level, etc. Nocturnal ventilation therapy, particularly with CPAP, is currently the treatment of first choice; numerous studies have confirmed its efficacy on symptoms (including daytime sleepiness), lung alterations, and cardiovascular changes, including vascular function.

In the last two decades there has been at least a fourfold increase in the prevalence of obesity, in particular of type III obesity, otherwise known as morbid obesity (BMI > 40 kg/m^2). Consequently, the number of patients affected by obesity-related respiratory disorders, in particular obesity-hypoventilation syndrome (OHS) is increasing. The term OHS has been used differently in the literature over the years. Initially it was coined to define patients with severe obesity, global respiratory failure, and severe hypoventilation/hypoxemia during sleep in the absence of episodes of obstructive apnea-hypopnea.

At present, the term is used to define obese patients (BMI ≥ 30 kg/m^2) with chronic alveolar hypoventilation, daytime hypercapnia (PaCO$_2$ ≥ 45 mmHg) and hypoxemia (PaO$_2$ < 70 mmHg), and respiratory disorders during sleep. In most cases (approximately 90 %) the respiratory disorder during sleep is OSA, while in the remaining 10 % the abnormality is frank, constant nocturnal hypoventilation with rare episodes of apnea or hypopnea (hourly apnea-hypopnea index <5 events/hour); in this case the patient must have a nighttime PaCO$_2$ value at least 10 mmHg higher than the value recorded while awake. Finally, it must be remembered that there are some patients with OSAS (an estimated 7 % of these patients) but with a BMI < 30 kg/m^2 who have daytime hypercapnia.

The few data available, generally derived from retrospective series, show a net increase in the prevalence of OHS with increasing BMI; the estimated prevalence in patients with a BMI > 40 kg/m^2 is approximately 25 %. These patients are responsible for greater healthcare resource consumption and have a higher mortality rate compared to subjects of the same weight without hypercapnia. A German study by Budweiser showed that ventilation treatment of OHS significantly reduced the 18-month mortality rate (Budweiser et al. 2007), while a French study showed that the 5-years mortality rate of OHS treated with NIV was 18.5 % (Prioux et al. 2010).

Recently, a subtype of Obesity-Hypoventilation Syndrome has been identified in extremely obese patients who had hypercapnic respiratory failure and multi-organ system dysfunction related to obesity: this condition has been called malignant obesity-hypoventilation syndrome (MOHS) (Marik and Desai 2013). In a retrospective review of the clinical data of 61 patients admitted to the ICU for hypercapnic respiratory failure with a BMI > 40 kg/m2 and a PaCO$_2$ > 45 mm Hg: 86 % of these patients had congestive heart failure treated with diuretics,

71 % had left ventricular failure, 61 % had left ventricular diastolic dysfunction, 77 % had pulmonary hypertension > 45 mm Hg, 90 % had essential hypertension, and 64 % had abnormal liver function tests and were diagnosed with nonalcoholic steatohepatitis. Although all these patients fitted the clinical criteria for OHS, before admission to the intensive care unit, only 3 were diagnosed with this condition and the remaining were diagnosed with and treated for chronic obstructive lung disease.

The pathophysiological mechanisms causing the development of chronic hypercapnia in a proportion of obese patients have not be completely clarified; Fig. 23.2 summarizes the most important mechanisms.

The state of obesity causes important changes to respiratory function. In the first place it has been described that lung volumes are redistributed with increasing weight. In detail, vital capacity and total lung capacity appear to be reduced only in the presence of a high BMI, while functional residual capacity and, above all, expiratory reserve volume are more compromised. The reduction in these latter volumes predisposes to a limitation of expiratory flow, which has been documented in these patients particularly when they are supine, an increase in the resistance of the lower airways and mismatching in the ventilation/perfusion ratio. The overall compliance of the respiratory system seems to be compromised by the reduced compliance of both the lungs (perhaps related to the greater volume of blood within the lungs) and the chest cage. The increases in both the elastic and non-elastic loads cause a net increment in respiratory work which is associated with inefficiency of the respiratory muscles, both for mechanical reasons essentially due to the mass of visceral fat and because of fatty infiltration within the muscles. In fact it has been demonstrated that the respiratory load is significantly greater in obese patients than in control subjects and, at the same time, that the

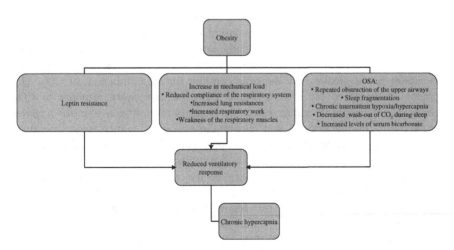

Fig. 23.2 Pathophysiological mechanisms hypothesized to be responsible for the development of chronic diurnal hypercapnia in obese subjects

respiratory work of hypoventilated obese patients is more than double that of patients with the same BMI but without hypercapnia.

The role of OSA in causing daytime hypercapnia was carefully examined by a group from New York in an important series of studies (Ayappa et al. 2002; Berger et al. 2000, 2002; Norman et al. 2006). In brief, this group demonstrated that the global minute volume does not decrease, or even increases, in patients with OSAS and daytime hypercapnia because of the marked hyperventilation after the apneic or hypopneic events. However, a progressive accumulation of CO_2 occurs as the ratio between the duration of the respiratory event and the phase of hyperventilation increases starting from 3:1; in these conditions the wash-out of the CO_2 accumulated during the phase of apnea/hypopnea is incomplete. The minute volume at the end of the obstructive event is closely associated with the accumulation of CO_2 during the event itself and is the main defense mechanism against the development of chronic hypercapnia in patients with OSA. In fact, these authors observed an inverse relationship between the slope of the post-event ventilatory response (ratio between the ventilatory response and CO_2 accumulation during the respiratory event) and the CO_2 level measured during wakefulness ($r = 0.90$, $p < 0.001$), suggesting that this mechanism of compensation is altered in some way in OSA patients with chronic hypercapnia. Obviously, the level of BMI plays a very important adjuvant role, negatively influencing both the accumulation of CO_2 during the event as well as the capacity for wash-out after the event. However, although the foregoing explains fairly well why a patient with OSAS, especially if obese, accumulates CO_2 during the hours of sleep, it does not provide a complete explanation for why chronic hypercapnia develops. The same research group offered a potential explanation in a study published in the *Journal of Applied Physiology* (Norman et al. 2006), hypothesizing a possible interaction between the respiratory and renal systems. Using an experimental model of the kinetics of CO_2, the authors simulated intermittent cycles of hypoxia and hypercapnia lasting 8 h (resembling the typical situation in a patient with OSA) repeated for 20 days. The progressive accumulation of CO_2 during the night caused an increase, albeit modest, in serum bicarbonate which the kidney was not able to deal with before the next period of sleep, given that the excretion time constant for bicarbonate was greater than the time constant for the elimination of CO_2. The gradual build up of bicarbonate would limit the ventilatory response to CO_2 compared to the initial value, since the changes in hydrogen ions for a given variation in CO_2 are reduced, thus resulting in a progressive increase in the values of CO_2. This reduction in ventilatory response to CO_2 is manifested during sleep also as the hyperventilation at the end of an obstructive respiratory event.

The validity of this hypothesis was recently confirmed by Raurich et al. in a group of 25 patients with OHS admitted to an intensive care unit for acute hypercapnic respiratory failure that required invasive mechanical ventilation for hypercapnic encephalopathy or failure of non invasive or invasive mechanical ventilation (Raurich et al. 2010). Patients with higher plasma bicarbonate had a more blunted CO_2 response than did those with lower plasma bicarbonate: BMI was not related to CO_2 response. Acetazolamide therapy, prescribed in patients with higher plasma bicarbonate, decreased the plasma bicarbonate and increased both the hypercapnic drive and hypercapnic ventilator response.

In conclusion, the most recently published data clearly show that the widespread opinion that patients with OSAS have normal respiratory function *a priori* must be corrected. It, therefore, seems obvious that an evaluation of respiratory function should always be included in the diagnostic protocols for OSA.

Suggested Reading

Ambrogio C, Koebnick J, Quan SF, Ranieri VM, Parthasarathy S (2008) Assessment of sleep in ventilator-supported critically ill patients. Sleep 31(11):1559–1568

Appelberg J, Pavlenko T, Bergman H et al (2007) Lung aeration during sleep. Chest 131(1):122–129

Ayappa I, Berger KI, Norman RG et al (2002) Hypercapnia and ventilatory periodicity in obstructive sleep apnea syndrome. Am J Respir Crit Care Med 166(8):1112–1115

Ballard RD, Clover CW, Suh BY (1995) Influence of sleep on respiratory function in emphysema. Am J Respir Crit Care Med 151(4):945–951

Becker HF, Piper AJ, Flynn WE et al (1999) Breathing during sleep in patients with nocturnal desaturation. Am J Respir Crit Care Med 159(1):112–118

Bednarek M, Plywaczewski R, Jonczak L, Zielinski J (2005) There is no relationship between chronic obstructive pulmonary disease and obstructive sleep apnea syndrome: a population study. Respiration 72(2):142–149

Berger KI, Ayappa I, Sorkin IB et al (2000) CO(2) homeostasis during periodic breathing in obstructive sleep apnea. J Appl Physiol 88(1):257–264

Berger KI, Ayappa I, Sorkin IB et al (2002) Postevent ventilation as a function of CO(2) load during respiratory events in obstructive sleep apnea. J Appl Physiol 93(3):917–924

Boyko Y, Ørding H, Jennum P (2012) Sleep disturbances in critically ill patients in ICU: how much do we know? Acta Anaesthesiol Scand 56:950–958

Bradley TD, Rutherford R, Lue F et al (1986) Role of diffuse airway obstruction in the hypercapnia of obstructive sleep apnea. Am Rev Respir Dis 134(5):920–924

Bradley TD, Mateika J, Li D et al (1990) Daytime hypercapnia in the development of nocturnal hypoxemia in COPD. Chest 97(2):308–312

Breslin E, van der Schans C, Breukink S et al (1998) Perception of fatigue and quality of life in patients with COPD. Chest 114(4):958–964

Budweiser S, Riedl SG, Jörres RA et al (2007) Mortality and prognostic factors in patients with obesity-hypoventilation syndrome undergoing noninvasive ventilation. J Intern Med 261(4):375–383

Catterall JR, Douglas NJ, Calverly PM et al (1983) Transient hypoxemia during sleep in chronic obstructive pulmonary disease is not a sleep apnea syndrome. Am Rev Respir Dis 128(1):24–29

Chan CS, Bye PT, Woolcock AJ, Sullivan CE (1990) Eucapnia and hypercapnia in patients with chronic airflow limitation. Am Rev Respir Dis 141(4 Pt 1):861–865 (The role of the upper airway)

Chaouat A, Weitzenblum E, Krieger J et al (1995) Association of chronic obstructive pulmonary disease and sleep apnea syndrome. Am J Respir Crit Care Med 151(1):82–86

Chaouat A, Weitzenblum E, Kessler R et al (1997) Sleep-related O_2 desaturation and daytime pulmonary haemodynamics in COPD patients with mild hypoxaemia. Eur Respir J 10(8):1730–1735

Chaouat A, Weitzenblum E, Kessler R et al (1999) A randomized trial of nocturnal oxygen therapy in chronic obstructive pulmonary disease patients. Eur Respir J 14(5):1002–1008

Chaouat A, Weitzenblum E, Kessler R et al (2001) Outcome of COPD patients with mild daytime hypoxaemia with or without sleep-related oxygen desaturation. Eur Respir J 17(5):848–855

Chapman KR, Mannino DM, Soriano JB et al (2006) Epidemiology and costs of chronic obstructive pulmonary disease. Eur Respir J 27(1):188–207

Connaughton JJ, Catterall JR, Elton RA et al (1988) Do sleep studies contribute to the management of patients with severe chronic obstructive pulmonary disease? Am Rev Respir Dis 138(2):341–344

Douglas NJ, Calverley PM, Leggett RJ et al (1979) Transient hypoxaemia during sleep in chronic bronchitis and emphysema. Lancet 1(8106):1–4

Drouot X, Roche-Campo F, Thille AW, Cabello B, Galia F, Margarit L, d'Ortho MP, Brochard L (2012) A new classification for sleep analysis in critically ill patients. Sleep Med 13(1):7–14

Dunroy HM, Adams L, Corfield DR, Morrell MJ (2003) CO_2 retention in lung disease; could there be a pre-existing difference in respiratory physiology. Respir Physiol Neurobiol 136(2–3):179–186

Fanfulla F, Grassi M, Taurino AE et al (2008) The relationship of daytime hypoxemia and nocturnal hypoxia in obstructive sleep apnea syndrome. Sleep 31(2):249–255

Fanfulla F, Ceriana P, D'Artavilla Lupo N, Trentin R, Frigerio F, Nava S (2011) Sleep disturbances in patients admitted to a step-down unit after ICU discharge: the role of mechanical ventilation. Sleep 34:355–362

Fleetham J, West P, Mezon B et al (1982) Sleep, arousals, and oxygen desaturation in chronic obstructive pulmonary disease. Am Rev Respir Dis 126(3):429–433

Flenley DC (1985) Sleep in chronic obstructive lung disease. Clin Chest Med 6(4):651–661

Fletcher EC, Miller J, Divine GW et al (1987) Nocturnal oxyhemoglobin desaturation in COPD patients with arterial oxygen tensions above 60 mmHg. Chest 92(4):604–608

Fletcher EC, Scott D, Qian W et al (1991) Evolution of nocturnal oxyhemoglobin desaturation in patients with chronic obstructive pulmonary disease and a daytime PaO_2 above 60 mmHg. Am Rev Respir Dis 144(2):401–405

Fletcher EC, Donner CF, Midgren B et al (1992) Survival in COPD patients with a daytime PaO_2 greater than 60 mmHg with and without nocturnal oxyhemoglobin desaturation. Chest 101(3):649–655

Flick MR, Bloch AJ (1977) Continuous in vivo monitoring of arterial oxygenation in chronic obstructive lung disease. Ann Intern Med 86(6):725–730

Freedman DS, Khan LK, Serdula MK et al (2002) Trends and correlates of class 3 obesity in the United States from 1990 through 2000. JAMA 288(14):1758–1761

Gòrecka D, Gorzelak K, Sliwinski P et al (1997) Effect of long-term oxygen therapy on survival in patients with chronic obstructive pulmonary disease with moderate hypoxaemia. Thorax 52(8):674–679

Guilleminault C, Cummiskey J, Motta J (1980) Chronic obstructive airflow disease and sleep studies. Am Rev Respir Dis 122(3):397–406

Hudgel DW, Martin RJ, Johnson B, Hill P (1984) Mechanics of the respiratory system and breathing pattern during sleep in normal humans. J Appl Physiol 56(1):133–137

Iber C, Ancoli-Israel S, Chesson AL, Quan SF (2007) The AASM manual for the scoring of sleep and associated events: rules, terminology, and technical specifications, 1st edn. American Academy of Sleep Medicine, Westchester

Jennum P, Riha RL (2009) Epidemiology of sleep apnoea/hypopnoea syndrome and sleep-disordered breathing. Eur Respir J 33(4):907–914

Johnson MW, Remmers JE (1984) Accessory muscle activity during sleep in chronic obstructive pulmonary disease. J Appl Physiol 57(4):1011–1017

Jones RL, Nzekwu MM (2006) The effects of body mass index on lung volumes. Chest 130(3):827–833

Koo KW, Sax DS, Snider GL (1975) Arterial blood gases and pH during sleep in chronic obstructive pulmonary disease. Am J Med 58(5):663–670

Laaban JP, Chailleux E (2005) Daytime hypercapnia in adult patients with obstructive sleep apnea syndrome in France, before initiating nocturnal nasal continuous positive airway pressure therapy. Chest 127(3):710–715

Larsson LG, Lindberg A, Franklin KA et al (2001) Obstructive sleep apnoea syndrome is common in subjects with chronic bronchitis. Respiration 68(3):250–255 (Reports from the Obstructive Lung Disease in Northern Sweden studies)

Leitch AG, Clancy LJ, Leggett RJ et al (1976) Arterial blood gas tensions, hydrogen ion, and electroencephalogram during sleep in patients with chronic ventilatory failure. Thorax 31(6):730–735

Levine S, Kaiser L, Leferovich J, Tikunov B (1997) Cellular adaptations in the diaphragm in chronic obstructive pulmonary disease. N Engl J Med 337(25):1799–1806

Levi-Valensi P, Weitzenblum E, Rida Z et al (1992) Sleep-related oxygen desaturation and daytime pulmonary haemodynamics in COPD patients. Eur Respir J 5(3):301–307

Lewis CA, Eaton TE, Fergusson W et al (2003) Home overnight pulse oximetry in patients with COPD: more than one recording may be needed. Chest 123(4):1127–1133

Little SA, Elkholy MM, Chalmers GW et al (1999) Predictors of nocturnal oxygen desaturation in patients with COPD. Respir Med 93(3):202–207

Macgowan NA, Evans KG, Road JD, Reid WD (2001) Diaphragm injury in individuals with airflow obstruction. Am J Respir Crit Care Med 163(7):1654–1659

Machado MCL, Vollmer VM, Togeiro SM, Bilderback AL, Oliveira MVC, Leitao FS, Queiroga F Jr, Lorenzi-Filho G, Krishnane JA (2010) CPAP and survival in moderate-to-severe obstructive sleep apnoea syndrome and hypoxaemic COPD. Eur Respir J 35:132–137

Marik PE, Desai H (2013) Characteristics of patients with the "Malignant Obesity Hypventilation Syndrome" admitted to an ICU. J Intensive Care 28(2):124–130

Marin JM, Soriano JB, Carrizo SJ, Boldoval A, Celli BR (2010) Outcomes in patients with chronic obstructive pulmonary disease and obstructive sleep apnea: the overlap syndrome. Am J Respir Crit Care Med 182:325–331

Marshall NS, Barnes M, Travier N et al (2006) Continuous positive airway pressure reduces daytime sleepiness in mild to moderate obstructive sleep apnoea: a meta-analysis. Thorax 61(5):430–434

McNicholas WT (2000) Impact of sleep in COPD. Chest 117(Suppl 2):48S–53S

Mokhlesi B, Kryger MH, Grunstein RR (2008) Assessment and management of patients with obesity hypoventilation syndrome. Proc Am Thorac Soc 5(2):218–225

Mulloy E, McNicholas WT (1993) Theophylline improves gas exchange during rest, exercise, and sleep in severe chronic obstructive pulmonary disease. Am Rev Respir Dis 148(4 Pt 1):1030–1036

Mulloy E, McNicholas WT (1996) Ventilation and gas exchange during sleep and exercise in severe COPD. Chest 109(2):387–394

Mutlu GM, Rubinstein I (2005) The saga of obstructive sleep apnea syndrome and daytime hypercapnia: work in progress. Chest 127(3):698–699

Norman RG, Goldring RM, Clain JM et al (2006) Transition from acute to chronic hypercapnia in patients with periodic breathing: predictions from a computer model. J Appl Physiol 100(5):1733–1741

O'Donoghue FJ, Catchside PG, Ellis EE et al (2003) Sleep hypoventilation in hypercapnic chronic obstructive pulmonary disease: prevalence and associated factors. Eur Respir J 21(6):977–984

O'Donoghue FJ, Catchside PG, Ecker DJ, McEvoy RD (2004) Changes in respiration in NREM sleep in hypercapnic chronic obstructive pulmonary disease. J Physiol 559(Pt 2):663–673

Plywaczewski R, Sliwinski P, Nowinski A et al (2000) Incidence of nocturnal desaturation while breathing oxygen in COPD patients undergoing long-term oxygen therapy. Chest 117(3):679–683

Poole DC, Sexton WL, Farkas GA et al (1997) Diaphragm structure and function in health and disease. Med Sci Sports Exerc 29(6):738–754

Prioux P, Hamel JF, Person C, Meslier N, Racineux JL, Urban T, Gagnadoux F (2010) Long-term outcome of noninvasive positive pressure ventilation for obesity hypoventilation syndrome. Chest 138(1):84–90

Raurich JM, Rialp G, Ibanez J, Llompart-Pou JA, Ayestaran J (2010) Hypercapnic respiratory failure in obesity-hypoventilation syndrome: CO_2 response and acetazolamide treatment effects. Respir Care 55(11):1442–1448

Reid WD, Samrai B (1995) Respiratory muscle training for patients with chronic obstructive pulmonary disease. Phys Ther 75(11):996–1005

Resta O, Foschino-Barbaro MP, Bonfitto P et al (2000) Prevalence and mechanisms of diurnal hypercapnia in a sample of morbidly obese subjects with obstructive sleep apnoea. Respir Med 94(3):240–246

Sajkov D, McEvoy RD (2009) Obstructive sleep apnea and pulmonary hypertension. Prog Cardiovasc Dis 51(5):363–370

Sandek K, Andersson T, Bratel T et al (1999) Sleep quality, carbon dioxide responsiveness and hypoxaemic patterns in nocturnal hypoxaemia due to chronic obstructive pulmonary disease (COPD) without daytime hypoxemia. Respir Med 93(2):79–87

Sanders MH, Newman AB, Haggerty CL et al (2003) Sleep and sleep-disordered breathing in adults with predominantly mild obstructive airway disease. Am J Respir Crit Care Med 167(1):7–14

Sergi M, Rizzi M, Andreoli A et al (2002) Are COPD patients with nocturnal REM sleep-related desaturations more prone to developing chronic respiratory failure requiring long-term oxygen therapy? Respiration 69(2):117–122

Sliwinski P, Macklem PT (1997) Inspiratory muscle dysfunction as a cause of death in COPD patients. Monaldi Arch Chest Dis 52(4):380–383

Stradling JR, Lane DJ (1983) Nocturnal hypoxaemia in chronic obstructive pulmonary disease. Clin Sci (Lond) 64:213–222

Tabachnick E, Muller NL, Bryan AC, Levison H (1981) Changes in ventilation and chest wall mechanics during sleep in normal adolescents. J Appl Physiol 51(3):557–564

Toraldo DM, Nicolardi G, De Nuccio F et al (2005) Pattern of variables describing desaturator COPD patients, as revealed by cluster analysis. Chest 128(6):3828–3837

Trask CH, Cree EM (1962) Oximeter studies on patients with chronic obstructive emphysema, awake and during sleep. N Engl J Med 266:639–642

Veale D, Chailleux E, Taytard A, Cardinaud JP (1998) Characteristics and survival of patients prescribed long-term oxygen therapy outside prescription guidelines. Eur Respir J 12(4):780–784

Vos PJ, Folgering HT, van Herwaarden CL (1995) Predictors for nocturnal hypoxaemia (mean $SaO_2 < 90\%$) in normoxic and mildly hypoxic patients with COPD. Eur Respir J 8(1):74–77

Wang D, Piper AJ, Wong KK et al (2011) Slow wave sleep in patients with respiratory failure. Sleep Med 12:378–383

White JE, Drinnan MJ, Smithson AJ et al (1995) Respiratory muscle activity and oxygenation during sleep in patients with muscle weakness. Eur Respir J 8(5):807–814

Nocturnal Ventilation: When to Use CPAP, When NIV

24

The therapeutic options for respiratory disorders during sleep have increased greatly in recent years. In the past the only treatment possibilities available were continuous positive pressure ventilation (CPAP) ventilation and bilevel pressure ventilation. Over the years other methods of ventilation have gradually been introduced, such as automatic CPAP, or auto-CPAP, average volume-assured pressure support (AVAPS), intelligent volume-assured pressure support (iVAPS), adaptive servo-ventilation (ASV), auto-bilevel ventilation (auto BiPAP) up to the most recent ones, auto-variable positive airway pressure (auto-VPAP or tri-level ventilation) or the TA-mode (automatic auto-adaptive).

Some of the methods of ventilation listed above lend themselves to widespread use for many disorders, whereas others has been introduced for selective use in some pathological states. Here, we shall consider the most common pathological conditions.

24.1 Obstructive Sleep Apnea Syndrome

The choice of treatment for obstructive sleep apnea syndrome (OSAS) depends on various factors, with the severity of the sleep-related respiratory changes and the presence of any comorbid conditions and their severity being particularly important.

The first-choice treatment for OSAS is definitely CPAP non invasive mechanical ventilation. There is a substantial body of scientific literature demonstrating the positive effects of this therapy, although at the same time highlighting its limitations and difficulty of use. The indications for this treatment, the ways to identify candidates for its use and the procedures for delivering the treatment have been defined by various national and international documents.

The indications for ventilation therapy with CPAP are:

- patients with a respiratory disturbance index (RDI) > 30 events/hour, independently of the presence of symptoms;

S. Nava and F. Fanfulla, *Non Invasive Artificial Ventilation*,
DOI: 10.1007/978-88-470-5526-1_24, © Springer-Verlag Italia 2014

- patients with an RDI of 5–30 events/hour, with symptoms of daytime sleepiness, impaired cognitive function, insomnia, and cardiovascular disorders.

The main mechanism of action of CPAP ventilation is very simple. It acts as a pneumatic splint by increasing the pressure within the upper airways to a level above their closure pressure, thus preventing the airways from collapsing. This form of ventilation is applied via an interface which can be one of the various types of mask, but is usually a nasal or oronasal mask. Other therapeutic strategies are to increase lung volumes, reduce edema of the upper airways, a more efficient system of controlling breathing and remodeling of the dilating muscles of the pharynx with normalization of their function.

There is now finally solid evidence that treatment with CPAP is effective in correcting the respiratory changes during sleep, reducing daytime sleepiness, and improving the patient's overall function, quality of life, and cognitive performance. Recent metaanalyses have compared the therapeutic effects of CPAP with those obtained with other treatments modalities, including intra-oral prostheses, conservative treatment, and placebo. In all cases the authors concluded by confirming the superiority of CPAP in obtaining optimal, global control of the disorder (Giles 2006, Guest 2008, McDaid 2009, Tan 2008).

The studies published in the literature generally document an improvement in all the polysomnographic indices, such as the apnea-hypopnea index (AHI), oxygen desaturation index (ODI), and the mean level of oxyhemoglobin saturation, compared with the results obtained with conservative treatment, positional management, or placebo, with further confirmation in the subsequent follow-ups (Giles 2006, Patel 2003). Likewise, CPAP did not have a negative affect on the duration of sleep compared with the results after administration of placebo or positional therapy; indeed, it actually produced a detectable improvement in the macrostructure of sleep through an increase in the percentage of slow wave and REM sleep and a reduction in the number of arousals. Obviously, the results depend strongly on the baseline level of impairment.

The effects of CPAP on the level of sleepiness and functional state are very complex as indeed are the methods used to measure these parameters. The impact of CPAP ventilation therapy on the level of somnolence, both objective and subjective, is usually evaluated by the Epworth sleepiness scale (ESS) proposed by Johns. Some studies, including one by Ballester, reported an improvement in the ESS score in subjects undergoing ventilation therapy compared to that in a group of patients treated with conservative therapy, including both sleep hygiene and weight loss (Ballester et al. 1999). A metaanalysis of all randomized, controlled studies published since 2001 on patients with excessive daytime sleepiness being treated with CPAP demonstrated that ventilation therapy significantly improves the objectively and subjectively determined level of sleepiness, reducing the ESS score, and increasing the latency before sleep. These results were most evident in subjects with the greatest impairment and with the most marked daytime sleepiness (ESS > 11) and were independent of age, body weight, and nationality. A subsequent metaanalysis, carried out considering seven randomized studies of subjects with mild-moderate OSA (AHI < 30 events/hour), demonstrated that treatment with CPAP led to a significant reduction in sleepiness, as evaluated by the ESS (mean reduction of 1.2 points) and an increase in vigilance (an increase in 2.1 min in the mean latency of falling asleep in the maintenance of wakefulness test). A randomized, controlled trial by Siccoli and colleagues added further confirmation of the improvement in the level of daytime sleepiness during treatment with CPAP, as well as an improvement in the quality of life (Siccoli et al. 2008).

There are still only limited data available on the efficacy of CPAP treatment on neurocognitive and psychological changes in patients with OSA. Two different studies, although performed by the same group, showed a significant improvement in the cognitive functions of patients undergoing CPAP treatment in comparison to those given a placebo. The data concerning improvements in other higher functions, such as attention, memory, and executive functions are contrasting (Giles 2006).

Recently, Antic et al. (2011) in a perspective study with a 3-months follow-up, demonstrated that a greater percentage of patients achieve normal functioning with a longer duration of use of nightly CPAP, but that neurobehavioral responses will not normalize in a substantial proportion of patients despite seemingly adequate CPAP use. The Authors concluded that is extremely important to assess patients carefully after CPAP therapy and to seek alternate etiologies and treatments for any residual abnormalities. Another similar study by Tomfohr et al. (2011), designed to assess the effect of CPAP on sleepiness and fatigue in patients with OSA, found that CPAP significantly reduced fatigue and increased energy as well as daytime sleepiness in patients who reported excessive sleepiness at the onset of treatment.

Similar considerations must be made regarding the impact of CPAP therapy on quality of life. The data available are not unequivocal, mainly because of the different assessment scales used. Some studies reported results in favor of CPAP, while other did not show significant differences between the effects of CPAP and the comparison treatments. Chronic treatment with CPAP seems to ensure an improvement in symptoms of depression, often observed in these patients.

The effects of CPAP therapy on cardiovascular disorders, in particular systemic hypertension, have been the subject of extensive research and numerous clinical trials (Becker, Cross, Pepperel). Some studies showed improvements in various factors and mechanisms involved in cardiovascular morbidity in patients with OSA, such as reductions in sympathetic tone, inflammation, markers of oxidative stress, and endothelial damage. CPAP therapy, in contrast to placebo, induces a significant improvement in systemic blood pressure; these results have been confirmed by a recent metaanalysis. Finally, other studies have demonstrated reductions in cardiovascular morbidity and mortality in patients with OSA being treated with CPAP. Recently, Sharma et al. (2011) in study designed to assess the impact of sleep apnea treatment on metabolic syndrome demonstrated that 3 months of CPAP therapy lowers blood pressure and partially reverses metabolic abnormalities. Furthermore, the impact of CPAP withdrawal on cardiovascular function in patients with moderate to severe OSA was evaluated by Kohler et al. (2011). The Authors found that CPAP withdrawal led to a rapid recurrence of OSA, a return of subjective sleepiness, and was associated with impaired endothelial function, increased urinary catecholamines, increased blood pressure, and faster heart rate.

24.1.1 Titration of CPAP

CPAP can be titrated in various ways, in accordance with the document produced by the Italian Association of Hospital Pulmonologists and the protocol proposed by the American Academy of Sleep Medicine (AASM):

- full, standard polysomnographic study with laboratory staff monitoring and manual adjustment of the CPAP values;
- full polysomnographic study, monitored or not, with the use of an auto-CPAP device;
- full polysomnographic study or full nocturnal cardiorespiratory monitoring during treatment with CPAP; the CPAP values are extrapolated from the auto-CPAP device used in the preceding nighttime registrations. The titration performed with an auto-CPAP device must be based on an analysis of a registration lasting at least 3–4 consecutive hours during which there must not be significant artifacts (leaks from the interface, detachment of the sensors).

The gold standard does, however, remain the full polysomnographic study and the therapeutic value of CPAP is defined as the minimum value of positive pressure able to correct the episodes of apnea, hypopnea, phasic oxygen desaturation, snoring, and micro-arousals related to the inspiratory flow limitation in all body positions and in all phases of sleep. The AASM proposes a less restrictive definition of the therapeutic value of CPAP, introducing three different levels of result:

1. Optimal titration—this reduces the RDI to values lower than 5 events/hour in a recording of at least 15 min, which includes a period of REM phase sleep in a supine position not interrupted by frequent arousals;
2. Good titration—reduces the global RDI (this refers to the whole night) to values ≤10 or to at least 50 % in cases in which the baseline value was <15; the recording must include at least a period of REM phase sleep in a supine position not interrupted by frequent arousals;
3. Adequate titration—persistence of global RDI >10 but less than 75 % of the baseline value, or meeting the criteria for optimal or good titration for the whole night, except the phases of REM sleep in a supine position.

Both documents reinforce the concept that the titration of CPAP in patients with concomitant disorders such as COPD, chronic heart failure, or neuromuscular diseases must be done during a full, standard polysomnographic study in a sleep laboratory.

24.1.2 Adherence to Treatment

Compliance with ventilation therapy is a key issue in the management of a patient with OSA. The final goal of the whole diagnostic and therapeutic process must be to achieve regular use of the ventilator. The optimal duration of treatment with CPAP during the night cannot be defined precisely because it depends on various factors, such as the different sleeping habits of the patients. However, use for less than 5 h/night is universally considered inadequate. The availability of new CPAP devices which include an internal memory system has made it possible to determine an individual patient's pattern of adherence to the therapeutic program and, if necessary, to plan personalized strategies to improve it. Patients with OSA actually seem to adhere to therapy considerably better than patients with other chronic disorders such as asthma, COPD (including oxygen therapy), or chronic heart disease. In real life about half of patients use CPAP every night for at least 6 h; the remaining patients either regularly use the ventilator for less than 6 h a night or allow themselves some pauses during the week (typically during the weekend). However, maintaining rigorous adherence to treatment seems to be extremely important because it is now clear that there is a sort of dose–response effect: the better the adherence to ventilation therapy, the greater the improvements that can be obtained. The minimum number of hours necessary to obtain therapeutic effects is not only subject to individual variability, but also depends on the outcome parameter considered: for example, in most patients use for more than 4 h achieves normalization of the subjective level of sleepiness, while more than 6 h use is necessary to obtain normalization of the level of sleepiness determined objectively.

Achieving an adequate level of adherence can be particularly difficult when the procedures of adaptation to ventilation therapy are limited or when the home-care system is not sufficiently involved in the education and follow-up of the patients. These aspects can explain the difference in compliance with CPAP treatment observed between American and European patients. In fact, the compliance with CPAP is systematically higher in Europe, generally being greater than 5 h/night.

Many studies have tried to identify possible factors that can influence, positively or negatively, compliance with treatment. Overall it can be stated that adherence is better in more severely affected patients, in those with greater sleepiness and in those who clearly perceive the clinical improvement. In contrast, there does not seem to be a direct relationship with the development of side effects. Finally, it has been clearly demonstrated that specific protocols of adaptation to treatment and educational support are critical factors for obtaining improved adherence to treatment. Early experience of telemedicine interventions promoted to improve CPAP adherence and to give adequate education and support is encouraging (Sparrow et al. 2010). The time passed between prescribing the ventilation therapy and the effective availability of the ventilator at the patient's home is equally important: the longer this time, the poorer the compliance will be. Finally, a psychological evaluation of the patient can help to identify his or her needs and expectations, integrating the standard education intervention with specific psycho-emotional and behavioral support.

24.1.3 Side Effects

Side effects of CPAP treatment are common: indeed approximately 60 % of patients report some type of problem with treatment, especially during the first few weeks.

The most commonly reported side effects are nasal congestion, dryness of the mucosae of the first part of the airways, and discomfort related to the flow of cold air. Episodes of epistaxis occur less frequently but can, sometimes, be severe, while the development of nasal congestion can compromise the continuation of treatment. The symptoms in the upper airways are usually caused by air leaks, mainly from mouth opening, which produces pronounced, one-directional flow from the nose to the oral mucosa. The development of these side effects can be prevented in various ways: use of a heated humidifier or greater care in the choice of the ventilation interface. Indeed, the quality of the mask is another equally critical factor, particularly for preventing the onset of oral respiration.

24.2   Persistence of OSA Despite CPAP Treatment

It is still possible to observe a substantial number of pathological respiratory events (apnea, hypopnea, desaturation events) in patients being treated with CPAP. Baltzan and colleagues performed a study with the aim of identifying the possible causes of persistent pathological events despite apparent correction of the disorder at the time of prescribing ventilation therapy (Baltzan et al. 2006). The prevalence of patients with persistent respiratory disorders was 17 % within the whole cohort of patients (n = 101) with a residual AHI >10 events/hour. These patients had a greater body mass index (BMI) at the time of diagnosis, required higher values of CPAP, showed more central-type events during the polysomnographic titration, needed more polysomnographic investigations for the titration of the CPAP and had greater problems of air leaks during the ventilation. Another 3-month follow-up study (Mulgrew et al. 2010) showed that the prevalence of persistent OSA despite careful CPAP titration was 25 %: the combination of downloaded data from the CPAP machine indicating a residual AHI > 10 events/h, together with residual sleepiness as evidenced by an ESS > 8, was the only predictor of persistent sleep apnea. Patients' outcomes including sleepiness (measured by ESS), quality of life (measured by the apnea quality of life index-SQALI), and CPAP compliance were worse for patients with residual sleep apnea compared with those without.

In recent years a problem known for many years, since the time that the only therapeutic option for OSAS was a permanent tracheotomy, has resurfaced. This problem is the development of repeated episodes of central apnea during ventilation therapy with CPAP that is effective in correcting the obstructive events. This phenomenon has been called complex sleep apnea syndrome, a term which should only be applied to those cases in which the patient has a typical picture of OSA, generally moderate or severe, at the baseline investigations and then, during treatment with CPAP, develops central events which are associated with desaturations and arousals. The few data available in the literature are heterogeneous. The prevalence of this condition varies between 6.5 and 15 %, although after a period of treatment with CPAP the prevalence seems to decrease to around 1.5 %. The different prevalence rates that have been published appear to be related to different percentages of patients with cardiac problems in the various cohorts of patients studied. In fact, the risk factors identified in these studies were influenced by the different populations investigated: Morgenthaler and colleagues did not identify any risk factors (Morgenthaler et al. 2006); male sex, a history of heart disease, and the presence of central-type sleep apnea in the baseline investigations were the risk factors that emerged from the work of Lehman and colleagues (2007), while Jahaveri and colleagues found that the severity of OSA, a central event index >5 at the baseline evaluation and the use of opioids were risk factors (Jahaveri et al. 2009).

24.2.1 Therapeutic Alternatives to CPAP During OSAS

There are essentially three possible alternatives to CPAP during OSAS. The first two, bilevel pressure ventilation and ventilation with auto-BiPAP, have been proposed for the treatment of patients with OSAS who require very high CPAP values, usually greater than $15–17$ cmH$_2$O, or those in whom CPAP treatment is not effective.

Bilevel pressure ventilation was conceived precisely with the aim of treating these patients; one possible approach to the titration of the ventilation parameters has been described thoroughly in the AASM guidelines, to which the reader is referred for full details (Kushida et al. 2008).

Ventilation with auto-BiPAP (*Respironics auto-BiPAP M series*®) was recently introduced with the purpose of enabling a more physiological treatment for those patients, often morbidly obese or with high compliance of the airways, who continue to manifest obstructive phenomena despite the use of high levels of positive pressure. This ventilator functions in a very physiological way, based on the principle that the obstructive events of the upper airways occur at different times in the respiratory cycle: the episodes of obstructive apnea or snoring usually start during expiration, whereas the episodes of hypopnea or inspiratory flow limitation are typically inspiratory events. This ventilator is, therefore, suitable for use in patients who require high levels of positive pressure or in patients who have major variability in obstructive events during the night, generally related to body position, phase of sleep, or variations in the resistance of the upper airways (e.g., changes in nasal resistance). The titration of the ventilation must, of course, be individualized and based on the data obtained in the previous nocturnal recording in which the failure of traditional CPAP treatment was demonstrated. The ventilator requires identification of a reference level of EPAP and a maximum level of IPAP; the operator must then set the maximum difference between the IPAP and EPAP. This ventilator is essentially able to modify the levels of expiratory and inspiratory pressures dynamically and separately depending on the patient's needs: the values of IPAP increase in the presence of hypopnea and inspiratory flow limitation, while the values of EPAP increase in the presence of apnea or snoring.

Finally, the third therapeutic alternative is ASV. This method, initially developed for the treatment of Cheyne-Stokes breathing in patients with chronic heart failure, has been used with relative success in patients with complex sleep apnea syndrome (Morgenthaler et al. 2007). It is currently difficult to foresee its systematic use, given the previously mentioned poor understanding of the pathophysiological mechanisms and the evolution over time of this particular form of OSAS. In fact, some patients with complex sleep apnea syndrome stabilize their own respiratory pattern after a period of treatment with traditional CPAP.

24.3 Obesity-Hypoventilation Syndrome

The therapeutic approach to this particular syndrome is complex. Ventilation treatment is the primary necessity in both acute and chronic cases. Figure 24.1 is a flow-chart showing the possible integrated therapeutic strategy.

The data in the literature show the marked efficacy of nocturnal ventilation therapy, whether with CPAP or NIV, in improving gas exchange and in controlling the state of chronic hypercapnia (Piper et al. 2008). As already mentioned, the main principle underlying the use of CPAP is to stabilize both the upper and lower airways, and improve the lung volumes. However, ventilation treatment with CPAP often does not seem sufficient either to control gas exchange during sleep, therefore necessitating the addition of oxygen therapy, or to control nocturnal hypoventilation adequately.

NIV is now widely used in these patients for the treatment of acute respiratory failure (when appropriate), as an alternative to invasive ventilation, for the prevention of re-intubation in patients previously treated invasively for an episode of acute respiratory failure, and for the treatment of chronic respiratory failure. The methods of ventilation used are the traditional ones, already described for acute respiratory failure, including AVAPS ventilation. At the moment there is not a standardized protocol for titrating the ventilation parameters. In the studies published so far, the level of EPAP is progressively increased until the obstructive events of the upper airways are corrected, while the level of IPAP is progressively increased to improve the minute volume (from the data available, the IPAP value is usually at least 8 cmH$_2$O higher than the EPAP). In a randomized, cross-over study comparing CPAP, BiPAP S/T, and AVAPS, Storre and colleagues demonstrated that NIV in a BiPAP mode produced substantial improvements in nocturnal oxygenation, sleep quality, and quality of life compared to CPAP treatment (Storre et al. 2006). Compared to the traditional BiPAP, ventilation in the AVAPS mode caused a further improvement in nocturnal ventilation with a more evident decrease in blood CO$_2$ levels. However, subsequent studies (Janssens et al. 2009; Carlucci et al. 2012) reported a greater sleep disruption as a consequence of the variation in inspiratory support delivered. A recent study, designed to investigate whether AVAPS ventilation is more effective in improving hypercapnia than fixed-level pressure support ventilation in patients with severe obesity, showed no differences between the two modes: at 3 months follow-up the mean changes in daytime arterial carbon dioxide was the same for both ventilation modes (Murphy et al. 2012).

In any case, independently of the mode of ventilation, it is known that the chronic use of NIV, like CPAP, improves lung volumes in these patients, mainly by increasing the expiratory reserve volume. Finally, in these patients too, the results are heavily dependent on the degree of adherence with the treatment, given that an improvement in blood gases can only be obtained with use for more than 5 h/night.

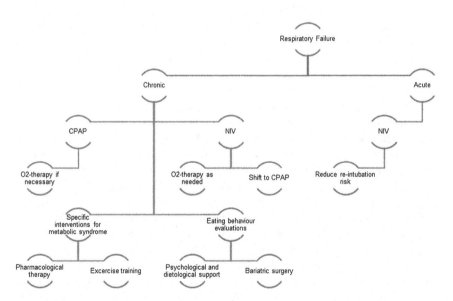

Fig. 24.1 Integrated therapeutic intervention for patients with obesity-hypoventilation syndrome and chronic respiratory failure

24.4 Alveolar Hypoventilation During Sleep

24.4.1 Procedures for Prescribing Long-Term NIV

Most patients receiving long-term NIV therapy, whether affected by COPD or restrictive chest disorders or neuromuscular diseases, receive their treatment while they are asleep. This choice is often also made for patients with chronic respiratory failure, and not only for those with respiratory disorders during sleep. The immediately noticeable result of NIV, especially when applied only during the nighttime hours, is an improvement in blood-gases while awake, which gives the patient more comfort and improves his or her quality of sleep.

The choice of the type of ventilation and its settings is a complex process. In normal clinical practice, the identification of the ventilator settings is based on an evaluation of the specific changes of respiratory function and the patient's level of comfort and is often made during a daytime trial, measuring the changes in blood-gases and the patient's tolerance of the therapy. However, the efficacy of mechanical ventilation set with this empirical approach has been demonstrated to be similar to that set on the basis of physiological criteria (i.e., a study of respiratory mechanics) only while the patient is awake.

The second phase, necessary for all patients undergoing nocturnal ventilation therapy is an evaluation of the efficacy of the treatment during sleep (whether during naps or nighttime sleep). There are various possible measurements, summarized in Table 24.1, but not all are commonly available in hospitals. In this regard it is important to emphasize the aim of nocturnal mechanical ventilation is not only to improve alveolar ventilation during sleep, but also, equally, to improve the patient's quality of sleep. In fact, independently of the underlying disease and its severity, little is currently known about the impact of ventilation therapy on the quality and structure of sleep or on the improvement of alveolar ventilation.

In fact it is known that patients with COPD or chronic respiratory failure can have various sleep alterations, such as reduced efficiency or marked fragmentation of sleep, a reduced percentage of slow-wave sleep or REM sleep, frequent body movements, and episodes of oxyhemoglobin desaturation. The few studies that have investigated the impact of long-term mechanical ventilation on sleep patterns have generally found an improvement in sleep structure compared to that observed during spontaneous breathing (Fig. 24.2). The factors that seem to influence the quality of sleep negatively during mechanical ventilation are the onset of changes in the respiratory pattern induced by the ventilation itself (for example, central apneas, periodic breathing), the choice of a ventilation method not appropriate for the patient's conditions, the presence of leaks from the mask, poor patient-ventilator coordination because of ineffective inspiratory efforts (Fig. 24.3), and phenomena of asynchrony in both the inspiratory and expiratory phases. The methods of titration used are determinant in the subsequent overall efficacy of the ventilation therapy. In fact, in a study that we carried out in patients with neuromuscular diseases already receiving long-term NIV, we showed that physiological titration

Table 24.1 Investigations for the diagnosis of the disease, determination of the degree of functional impairment, and setting the ventilation parameters

Test	Use	Limitations	Advantages
Measurement of lung volumes	Always necessary for correct functional diagnosis and to monitor deterioration in respiratory function		
Maximum respiratory pressures at the mouth	See above		
Respiratory pattern during spontaneous breathing	Important, but not essential		Provides a guide to the choice of ventilator settings
Respiratory pattern during ventilation while awake	Together with the blood-gas analysis enables an evaluation of the response to mechanical ventilation	Tidal volume can only be quantified by using plethysmographic techniques and calibration of volumes	Guides the choice of ventilator settings
Daytime arterial blood-gases	Essential, both in basal conditions and during ventilation	Only intermittent information on blood-gas status	Reference test for evaluating, during wakefulness, blood-gases and their changes during mechanical ventilation
Nocturnal polysomnography/ polygraphy	Essential for the correct diagnosis of sleep-related respiratory disorders	Does not identify the REM phases of sleep (limited to cardiorespiratory monitoring) Some systems do not use inductive plethysmography	Only method for evaluating the patient/ventilator interaction and identifying all the factors that limit the efficacy of mechanical ventilation
Nocturnal pulse oximetry	Exclusive evaluation of the state of nocturnal oxygenation	Cannot be used to evaluate the efficacy of the ventilation	Useful for titrating O_2 flow
Transcutaneous monitoring of blood-gases	Provides an evaluation of the trends in blood-gases	Measurements not always valid and stable (must be compared with blood-gas data), delay in the response of the sensors, side effects related to the sensors, expensive	Possibility of evaluating the degree of hypoventilation; evaluation of the response to ventilation therapy during sleep

(continued)

Table 24.1 (continued)

Test	Use	Limitations	Advantages
Respiratory mechanics	Very useful for physiological identification of ventilation parameters	Relatively invasive and complex; requires specific equipment	The ventilator settings are determined on the basis of the patient's specific mechanical requirements

(based on data from studies of respiratory mechanics) of the ventilation parameters was associated with better gas exchange during sleep, as well as better sleep quality, compared to empirical titration (essentially based on data collected while the patient was awake). Furthermore, the improvements in sleep quality were associated with a reduction in the number of ineffective inspiratory efforts

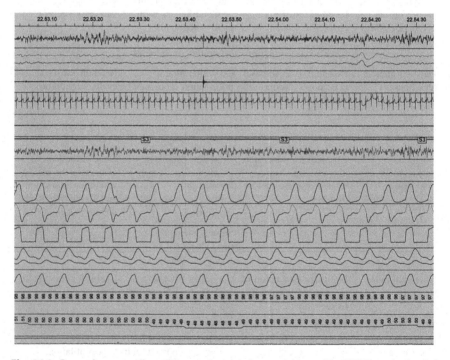

Fig. 24.2 Part of a recording (90-second strip) in a patient with COPD and alveolar hypoventilation during sleep. Note the excellent coordination between the patient and the ventilator. The signals recorded are (from the *top* downwards): electroencephalogram (C_4–A_1), *left* and *right* electro-oculograms; submental electromyogram; *left* and *right* anterior tibial electromyograms; electrocardiogram; electroencephalogram (C_3–A_2); microphone; tidal volume; air flow; pressure in the mask; thoracic and abdominal respirograms (with inductive plethysmography); sum of thoracic and abdominal activity (plethysmographic method); SpO_2; heart rate; body position

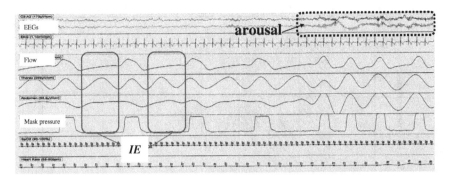

Fig. 24.3 A 60-second section of a recording in a patient with COPD receiving ventilation therapy with NIV. Note the repeated ineffective inspiratory efforts (*IE*) that induce arousal reactions. The signals recorded, from top downwards, are: electroencephalogram (C_4–A_1; C_3–A_2), electrocardiogram; microphone; airflow; chest and abdominal respirograms (with inductive plethysmography); pressure in the mask; SpO_2; heart rate

(Fanfulla et al. 2005). In a subsequent study, we investigated the prevalence of patient/ventilator asynchrony in a group of patients (n = 48) with other chronic diseases, COPD, obesity-hypoventilation, or kyphoscoliosis, already receiving home ventilation treatment (Fanfulla et al. 2007). In the first place, although none of the patients had ineffective inspiratory efforts while awake, only four patients had fewer than 5 ineffective efforts/hour during sleep (Fig. 24.4); indeed, the mean number of ineffective efforts was 48 ± 39.5, without appreciable differences between patients grouped according to the underlying disorder that had caused the respiratory failure. Finally, the presence of ineffective inspiratory efforts was associated with a worsening of nocturnal gas exchange. Subsequent studies confirmed these results, demonstrating that the setting of ventilation parameters in patients with nocturnal hypoventilation must be made during sleep or, at least, a nocturnal verification (polysomnographic or polygraphic) must be made of the efficacy of the parameters set during wakefulness.

However, patients with chronic alveolar hypoventilation, independently of the underlying disease, may also have instability of the upper airways leading to apnea or hypopnea events. Furthermore, it is well-known that some patients being ventilated mechanically may develop (mainly during sleep) active glottic closure which is related to the changes in total ventilation or arterial CO_2. These events are characterized by a simultaneous reduction or abolition of inspiratory effort, probably reflecting a decrease in ventilatory command. Finally, clusters of periodic breathing or central apnea during sleep have been reported in patients receiving mechanical ventilation, invasively or non invasively, in both acute and chronic settings.

From this point of view, interesting developments could derive from the future use of new methods of ventilation that have recently become available, characterized by the possibility of varying the level of pressure support based on the

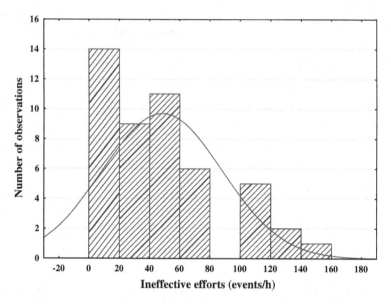

Fig. 24.4 Distribution of the hourly index of ineffective efforts during a nighttime recording. Reproduced from Fanfulla et al. 2007, with permission from Elsevier

patient's needs, or by the incorporation of systems to monitor patient-ventilator asynchrony in traditional ventilators (Mulqueeny et al. 2007).

Taking into account all the above, it is clear that the ventilator setting procedure in patients who are candidates for long-term mechanical ventilation is not "so easy", but requires specific organization, protocols, and equipment (Mandal et al. 2013).

The AASM identified best clinical practices for the sleep center adjustment of NIV in stable chronic alveolar hypoventilation syndromes, also providing a complete list of the technical equipment (Berry et al. 2010). The AASM protocol considers polysomnography as the recommended method to determine an effective level of nocturnal ventilatory support, or, when NIV treatment is initiated and adjusted empirically in the outpatient setting based on clinical judgment, to confirm that the final non invasive positive pressure ventilation settings are effective or to make adjustments as necessary.

A multicenter European work group (SomnoNIV) proposed standard classifications and definitions of some clinically relevant respiratory events that may occur during mechanical ventilation and a standard approach to identify these events during nocturnal recording (poligraphy or polysomnography (Gonzalez-Bermeio et al. 2012); however, phenomena of altered patients-ventilator interactions, such as ineffective efforts, double or auto-triggering, or hang-up, were not included.

The SomnoNIV group also reviewed the role and limits of simple techniques such as pulse oximetry, capnography, built-in ventilator software, and autonomic markers of sleep fragmentation to monitor or assess NIV efficacy during sleep (Janssens et al. 2011). They proposed an interesting algorithm largely based on clinical symptoms, daytime $PaCO_2$, nocturnal pulse oximetry, and data obtained by the built-in software that may help clinicians to identify those patients who require more complex procedures such as sleep studies.

One often neglected aspect that is able to influence the therapeutic results negatively is the choice of ventilator. A variety of studies have investigated different aspects of the performance of the mechanical ventilators commonly used for home ventilation, showing marked differences in technical parameters between the various models: sensitivity and speed of the trigger, pressurization time, coherence between the levels of positive pressure set and those actually supplied, etc. (Chatwin et al. 2010).

Finally, in the context of long-term treatment, the choice of the best interface, as well as the home management of the equipment, are of paramount importance. The range of possible interfaces to choose from is now very good, given the availability of various models of masks, nasal and oronasal interfaces, and systems derived from the Adams circuit. Published data have not shown significant differences between the various types of interfaces with regards to the extent of the improvement in blood-gases. The choice should, therefore, be guided by the patient on the basis of his or her preferences with the aim of reaching the best compromise among comfort, amount of air leakage, ease of use, and compatibility with the chosen home ventilator. The indication for associated oxygen should be assessed individually with the purpose of maintaining an adequate nocturnal level of SaO_2 (>92 %), but only after having optimized the ventilation settings.

Finally, once the home ventilation treatment has been started, its efficacy should be checked with a specific follow-up program, through measurements of daytime blood-gases, nocturnal respiratory function indices, or subjective indicators (quality of life, compliance, dyspnea, symptoms, etc.). There is substantial evidence, from studies carried out throughout the world, that home care programs of whatever type, provided that they are specifically designed for patients with COPD or chronic respiratory failure, improve patients' survival, reduce hospital admissions, including those to an intensive care unit, decrease the number of exacerbations and, therefore, in the final analysis, the costs of the chronic respiratory disease. It is, therefore, important to have a well-organized, global management model that may serve as a "reference" for each future care protocol designed for each local need (Veale et al. 2010).

Suggested Reading

Allam JS, Olson EJ, Gay PC, Morgenthaler TI (2007) Efficacy of adaptive servoventilation in treatment of complex and central sleep apnea syndromes. Chest 132(6):1839–1846

Antic NA, Catcheside P, Buchan C et al (2011) The effect of CPAP in normalizing daytime sleepiness, quality of life, and neurocognitive function in patients with moderate to severe OSA. Sleep 34(1):111–119

Bachour A, Maasilta P (2004) Mouth breathing compromises adherence to nasal continuous positive airway pressure therapy. Chest 126(4):1248–1254

Bachour A, Hurmerinta K, Maasilta P (2004) Mouth closing device (chinstrap) reduces mouth leak during nasal CPAP. Sleep Med 5(3):261–267

Ballester E, Badia JR, Hernàndez L et al (1999) Evidence of the effectiveness of continuous positive airway pressure in the treatment of sleep apnea/hypopnea syndrome. Am J Respir Crit Care Med 159(2):495–501

Baltzan MA, Kassissia I, Elkholi O et al (2006) Prevalence of persistent sleep apnea in patients treated with continuous positive airway pressure. Sleep 29(4):557–563

Baltzan MA, Elkholi O, Wolkove N (2009) Evidence of interrelated side effects with reduced compliance in patients treated with nasal continuous positive airway pressure. Sleep Med 10(2):198–205

Banerjee D, Yee BJ, Piper AJ et al (2007) Obesity hypoventilation syndrome: hypoxemia during continuous positive airway pressure. Chest 131(6):1678–1684

Basner RC (2007) Continuous positive airway pressure for obstructive sleep apnea. N Engl J Med 356(17):1751–1758

Battisti A, Tassaux D, Janssens JP et al (2005) Performance characteristics of 10 home mechanical ventilators in pressure-support mode: a comparative bench study. Chest 127(5):1784–1792

Becker HF, Jerrentrup A, Ploch T et al (2003) Effect of nasal continuous positive airway pressure treatment on blood pressure in patients with obstructive sleep apnea. Circulation 107(1):68–73

Berry RB, Chediak A, Brown LK, Finder J, Gozal D, Iber C, Kushida CA, Morgenthaler T, Rowley JA, Davidson-Ward SL (2010) Best clinical practices for the sleep center adjustment of noninvasive positive pressure ventilation (NPPV) in stable chronic alveolar hypoventilation syndromes. J Clin Sleep Med 6(5):497–509

Caples SM, Gami AS, Somers VK (2005) Obstructive sleep apnea. Ann Intern Med 142(3):187–197

Carlucci A, Fanfulla F, Mancini M, Nava S (2012) Volume assured pressure support ventilation—induced arousals. Sleep Med 13(6):767–768

Chatwin M, Heather S, Hanak A, Polkey MI, Simonds AK (2010) Analysis of home support and ventilator malfunction in 1211 ventilator-dependent patients. Eur Respir J 35:310–316

Consensus Conference (1999) Clinical indications for noninvasive positive pressure ventilation in chronic respiratory failure due to restrictive lung disease, COPD, and nocturnal hypoventilation: a consensus conference report. Chest 116(2):521–534

Cross MD, Mills NL, Al-Abri M et al (2008) Continuous positive airway pressure improves vascular function in obstructive sleep apnoea/hypopnoea syndrome: a randomised controlled trial. Thorax 63(7):578–583

D'Ambrosio C, Bowman T, Mohsenin V (1999) Quality of life in patients with obstructive sleep apnea: effect of nasal continuous positive airway pressure—a prospective study. Chest 115(1):123–129

Dellweg D, Barchfeld T, Klauke M, Eiger G (2009) Respiratory muscle unloading during autoadaptive non-invasive ventilation. Respir Med 193(11):1706–1712

Devouassoux G, Lévy P, Rossini E et al (2007) Sleep apnea is associated with bronchial inflammation and continuous positive airway pressure-induced airway hyperresponsiveness. J Allergy Clin Immunol 119(3):597–603

Dimsdale JE, Loredo JS, Profant J (2000) Effect of continuous positive airway pressure on blood pressure: a placebo trial. Hypertension 35(1 Pt 1):144–147

El-Solh AA, Aquilina A, Pineda L et al (2006) Noninvasive ventilation for prevention of postextubation respiratory failure in obese patients. Eur Respir J 28(3):588–595

Engleman HM, Martin SE, Deary IJ, Douglas NJ (1994) Effect of continuous positive airway pressure treatment on daytime function in sleep apnoea-hypopnea syndrome. Lancet 343(8897):572–575

Engleman HM, Kingshott RN, Wraight PK et al (1999) Randomized placebo-controlled crossover trial of continuous positive airway pressure for mild sleep apnoea/hypopnea syndrome. Am J Respir Crit Care Med 159(2):461–467

Faccenda JF, Mackay TW, Boon NA, Douglas NJ (2001) Randomized placebo-controlled trial of continuous positive airway pressure on blood pressure in the sleep apnea-hypopnea syndrome. Am J Respir Crit Care Med 163(2):344–348

Fanfulla F, Delmastro M, Berardinelli A et al (2005) Effects of different ventilator settings on sleep and inspiratory effort in patients with neuromuscular disease. Am J Respir Crit Care Med 172(5):619–624

Fanfulla F, Taurino AE, Lupo ND et al (2007) Effect of sleep on patient/ventilator asynchrony in patients undergoing chronic non-invasive mechanical ventilation. Respir Med 101(8):1702–1707

Gay PC, Hubmayr RD, Stroetz RW (1996) Efficacy of nocturnal nasal ventilation in stable, severe chronic obstructive pulmonary disease during a 3-month controlled trial. Mayo Clin Proc 71(6):533–542

Gay P, Weaver T, Loube D et al (2006) Evaluation of positive airway pressure treatment for sleep related breathing disorders in adults. Sleep 29(3):381–401

Giles TL, Lasserson TJ, Smith BJ et al (2006) Continuous positive airways pressure for obstructive sleep apnoea in adults. Cochrane Database Syst Rev (1):CD001106

Gonzalez-Bermeio J, Perrin C, Janssens JP et al (2012) Proposal for a systematic analysis of polygraphy or polysomnography for identifying and scoring abnormal events occurring during non-invasive ventilation. Thorax 67:546–552

Gonzàlez MM, Parreira VF, Rodenstein DO (2002) Non-invasive ventilation and sleep. Sleep Med Rev 6(1):29–44

Guest JF, Helter MT, Morga A, Stradling JR (2008) Cost-effectiveness of using continuous positive airway pressure in the treatment of severe obstructive sleep apnoea/hypopnoea syndrome in the UK. Thorax 63(10):860–865

Guo YF, Sforza E, Janssens JP (2007) Respiratory patterns during sleep in obesity-hypoventilation patients treated with nocturnal pressure support: a preliminary report. Chest 131(4):1090–1099

Haentjens P, Van Meerhaeghe A, Moscariello A et al (2007) The impact of continuous positive airway pressure on blood pressure in patients with obstructive sleep apnea syndrome: evidence from a meta-analysis of placebo-controlled randomized trials. Arch Intern Med 167(8):757–765

Haniffa M, Lasserson TJ, Smith I (2004) Interventions to improve compliance with continuous positive airway pressure for obstructive sleep apnoea. Cochrane Database Syst Rev 18(4):CD003531

Heinemann F, Budweiser S, Dobroschke J, Pfeifer M (2007) Non-invasive positive pressure ventilation improves lung volumes in the obesity hypoventilation syndrome. Respir Med 101(6):1229–1235

Hoy CJ, Vennelle M, Kingshott RN et al (1999) Can intensive support improve continuous positive airway pressure use in patients with the sleep apnea/hypopnea syndrome? Am J Respir Crit Care Med 159(4 Pt 1):1096–1100

Hui DS, Choy DK, Li TS et al (2001) Determinants of continuous positive airway pressure compliance in a group of Chinese patients with obstructive sleep apnea. Chest 120(1):170–176

Insalaco G, Sanna A, Fanfulla F et al (2005) La terapia con dispositivo a pressione positiva nelle vie aeree: raccomandazioni per la prescrizione nel soggetto adulto affetto dalla sindrome delle apnee ostruttive nel sonno. Documento dell'Associazione Italiana Pneumologi Ospedalieri (AIPO) a cura del gruppo di studio "Disturbi respiratori nel sonno". Available at: www.aiponet.it

Janssens JP, Metzger M, Sforza E (2009) Impact of volume targeting on efficacy of bi-level non-invasive ventilation and sleep in obesity-hypoventilation. Respir Med 103:165–172

Janssens JP, Borel JC, Pepin JL et al (2011) Nocturnal monitoring of home non-invasive ventilation: the contribution of simple tools such as pulse oximetry, capnography, built-in ventilator software and autonomic markers of sleep fragmentation. Thorax 66(5):438–445

Javaheri S, Smith J, Chung E (2009) The prevalence and natural history of complex sleep apnea. J Clin Sleep Med 5(3):205–211

Jaye J, Chatwin M, Dayer M et al (2009) Autotitrating versus standard noninvasive ventilation: a randomized crossover trial. Eur Respir J 33(3):566–571

Jones SE, Packham S, Hebden M, Smith AP (1998) Domiciliary nocturnal intermittent positive pressure ventilation in patients with respiratory failure due to severe COPD: long-term follow up and effect on survival. Thorax 53(6):495–498

Johns MW (1991) A new method for measuring daytime sleepiness: the Epworth sleepiness scale. Sleep 14(6):540–545

Kingshott RN, Vennelle M, Hoy CJ et al (2000) Predictors of improvements in daytime function outcomes with CPAP therapy. Am J Respir Crit Care Med 161(3 Pt 1):866–871

Kohler M, Stoewhas AC, Ayers L, Senn O, Bloch KE, Russi EW, Stradling JR (2011) Effects of continuous positive airway pressure therapy withdrawal in patients with obstructive sleep apnea. Am J Respir Crit Care Med 184:1192–1199

Kribbs NB, Pack AI, Kline LR et al (1993) Objective measurement of patterns of nasal CPAP use by patients with obstructive sleep apnea. Am Rev Respir Dis 147(4):887–895

Krieger J, McNicholas WT, Levy P et al (2002) Public health and medicolegal implications of sleep apnoea. Eur Respir J 20(6):1594–1609

Kushida CA, Littner MR, Hirshkowitz M et al (2006) Practice parameters for the use of continuous and bilevel positive airway pressure devices to treat adult patients with sleep-related breathing disorders. Sleep 29(3):375–380

Kushida CA, Chediak A, Berry RB et al (2008) Positive airway pressure titration task force of the American Academy of Sleep Medicine. Clinical guidelines for the manual titration of positive airway pressure in patients with obstructive sleep apnea. J Clin Sleep Med 4(2):157–171

Lehman S, Antic NA, Thompson C et al (2007) Central sleep apnea on commencement of continuous positive airway pressure in patients with a primary diagnosis of obstructive sleep apnea-hypopnea. J Clin Sleep Med 3(5):462–466

Linee Guida di Procedura Diagnostica nella Sindrome delle Apnee Ostruttive nel Sonno dell'Adulto. Commissione Paritetica Associazione Italiana Medicina del Sonno (AIMS) e Associazione Italiana Pneumologi Ospedalieri (AIPO). Available at www.aiponet.it or www.sonnomed.it

Loredo JS, Ancoli-Israel S, Dimsdale JE (1999) Effect of continuous positive airway pressure versus placebo continuous positive airway pressure on sleep quality in obstructive sleep apnoea. Chest 116(6):1545–1549

Mandal S, Suh E, Davies M et al (2013) Provision of home mechanical ventilation and sleep service for England survey. Thorax 68(9):880–881

Marin JM, Carrizo SJ, Vicente E, Agusti AG (2005) Long-term cardiovascular outcomes in men with obstructive sleep apnoea-hypopnoea with or without treatment with continuous positive airway pressure: an observational study. Lancet 365(9464):1046–1053

Marshall NS, Barnes M, Travier N et al (2006) Continuous positive airway pressure reduces daytime sleepiness in mild to moderate obstructive sleep apnoea: a meta-analysis. Thorax 61(5):430–434

Martins De Araùjo MT, Vieira SB, Vasquez EC, Fleury B (2000) Heated humidification or face mask to prevent upper airway dryness during continuous positive airway pressure therapy. Chest 117(1):142–147

Massie CA, Hart RW (2003) Clinical outcomes related to interface type in patients with obstructive sleep apnea/hypopnea syndrome who are using continuous positive airway pressure. Chest 123(4):1112–1118

Massie CA, Hart RW, Peralez K, Richards GN (1999) Effects of humidification on nasal symptoms and compliance in sleep apnea patients using continuous positive airway pressure. Chest 116(2):403–408

McDaid C, Griffin S, Weatherly H et al (2009) Continuous positive airway pressure devices for the treatment of obstructive sleep apnoea–hypopnoea syndrome: a systematic review and economic analysis. Health Technol Assess 13(4)

McNicholas WT, Bonsigore MR (2007) Sleep apnoea as an independent risk factor for cardiovascular disease: current evidence, basic mechanisms and research priorities. Eur Respir J 29(1):156–178

Meecham Jones DJ, Paul EA, Jones PW, Wedzicha JA (1995) Nasal pressure support ventilation plus oxygen compared with oxygen therapy alone in hypercapnic COPD. Am J Respir Crit Care Med 152(2):538–544

Mehta S, Hill NS (2001) Noninvasive ventilation. Am J Respir Crit Care Med 163(2):540–577

Mokhlesi B, Tulaimat A, Evans AT et al (2006) Impact of adherence with positive airway pressure therapy on hypercapnia in obstructive sleep apnea. J Clin Sleep Med 2(1):57–62

Monasterio C, Vidal S, Duran J et al (2001) Effectiveness of continuous positive airway pressure in mild sleep apnea-hypopnea syndrome. Am J Respir Crit Care Med 164(6):939–943

Morgenthaler TI, Kagramanov V, Hanak V, Decker PA (2006) Complex sleep apnea syndrome: is it a unique clinical syndrome? Sleep 29(9):1203–1209

Morgenthaler TI, Gay PC, Gordon N, Brown LK (2007) Adaptive servoventilation versus noninvasive positive pressure ventilation for central, mixed, and complex sleep apnea syndromes. Sleep 30(4):468–547

Morgenthaler TI, Aurora RN, Brown T et al (2008) Standards of Practice Committee of the AASM. Practice parameters for the use of autotitrating continuous positive airway pressure devices for titrating pressures and treating adult patients with obstructive sleep apnea syndrome: an update for 2007. An American Academy of Sleep Medicine report. Sleep 31(1):141–147

Mulgrew AT, Lawati NA, Ayas NT, Fox N, Hamilton P, Cortes L, Ryan CF (2010) Residual sleep apnea on polysomnography after 3 months of CPAP therapy: clinical implications, predictors and patterns. Sleep Med 11:119–125

Mulqueeny Q, Ceriana P, Carlucci A et al (2007) Automatic detection of ineffective triggering and double triggering during mechanical ventilation. Intensive Care Med 33(11):2014–2018

Murphy PB, Davidson C, Hind MD, Simonds A et al (2012) Volume targeted versus pressure support non-invasive ventilation in patients with super obesity and chronic respiratory failure: a randomised controlled trial. Thorax 67:727–734

Patel SR, White DP, Malhotra A et al (2003) Continuous positive airway pressure therapy for treating sleepiness in a diverse population with obstructive sleep apnea: results of a meta-analysis. Arch Intern Med 163(5):565–571

Patruno V, Aiolfi S, Costantino G et al (2007) Fixed and autoadjusting continuous positive airway pressure treatments are not similar in reducing cardiovascular risk factors in patients with obstructive sleep apnea. Chest 131(5):1393–1399

Pelletier-Fleury N, Meslier N, Gagnadoux F et al (2004) Economic arguments for the immediate management of moderate-to-severe obstructive sleep apnoea syndrome. Eur Respir J 23(1):53–60

Pépin JL, Leger P, Veale D et al (1995) Side effects of nasal continuous positive airway pressure in sleep apnea syndrome. Study of 193 patients in two French sleep centers. Chest 107(2):375–381

Pépin JL, Krieger J, Rodenstein D et al (1999) Effective compliance during the first 3 months of continuous positive airway pressure. A European prospective study of 121 patients. Am J Respir Crit Care Med 160(4):1124–1129

Peppard PE, Young T, Palta M, Skatrud J (2000) Prospective study of the association between sleep-disordered breathing and hypertension. N Engl J Med 342(19):1378–1384

Pepperell JC, Ramdassingh-Dow S, Crosthwaite N et al (2002) Ambulatory blood pressure after therapeutic and subtherapeutic nasal continuous positive airway pressure for obstructive sleep apnoea: a randomised parallel trial. Lancet 359(9302):204–210

Pierobon A, Giardini A, Fanfulla F et al (2008) A multidimensional assessment of obese patients with obstructive sleep apnoea syndrome (OSAS): a study of psychological, neuropsychological and clinical relationships in a disabling multifaceted disease. Sleep Med 9(8):882–889

Piper AJ, Wang D, Yee BJ, Barnes DJ, Grunstein RR (2008) Randomised trial of CPAP vs bilevel support in the treatment of obesity hypoventilation syndrome without severe nocturnal desaturation. Thorax 63:395–401

Poulet C, Veale D, Arnol N et al (2009) Psychological variables as predictors of adherence to treatment by continuous positive airway pressure. Sleep Med 10(9):993–999

Redline S, Adams N, Strauss ME et al (1998) Improvement of mild sleep-disordered breathing with CPAP compared with conservative therapy. Am J Respir Crit Care Med 157(3 Pt 1):858–865

Robert D, Argaud L (2007) Non-invasive positive ventilation in the treatment of sleep-related breathing disorders. Sleep Med 8(4):441–452

Schwartz DJ, Karatinos G (2007) For individuals with obstructive sleep apnea, institution of CPAP therapy is associated with an amelioration of symptoms of depression which is sustained long term. J Clin Sleep Med 3(6):631–635

Sharma SK, Agrawal S, Damodaran D et al (2011) CPAP for the metabolic syndrome in patients with obstructive sleep apnea. N Engl J Med 365:2277–2286

Siccoli MM, Pepperell JC, Kohler M et al (2008) Effects of continuous positive airway pressure on quality of life in patients with moderate to severe obstructive sleep apnea: data from a randomized controlled trial. Sleep 31(11):1551–1558

Sparrow D, Aloia M, DeMolles DA et al (2010) A telemedicine intervention to improve adherence to continuous positive airway pressure: a randomized controlled trial. Thorax 65:1061–1066

Storre JH, Seuthe B, Fiechter R et al (2006) Average volume-assured pressure support in obesity hypoventilation: a randomized crossover trial. Chest 130(3):815–821

Tan MCY, Ayas NT, Mulgrew A, Cortes L et al (2008) Cost-effectiveness of continuous positive airway pressure therapy in patients with obstructive sleep apnea-hypopnea in British Columbia. Can Respir J 15(3):159–165

Tobin MJ, Jubran A, Laghi F (2001) Patient-ventilator interaction. Am J Respir Crit Care Med 163(5):1059–1063

Tomfohr LM, Ancoli-Israel S, Loredo JS, Dimsdale JE (2011) Effects of continuous positive airway pressure on fatigue and sleepiness in patients with obstructive sleep apnea: data from a randomized controlled trial. Sleep 34(1):121–126

Veale D, Gonzalez-Bermejo J, Borel JC et al (2010) Initiation of long-term non-invasive ventilation at home: current practices and expected issues. Survey from the CasaVNI working party. Revue des Mal Respiratoire 27:1022–1029

Vitacca M, Nava S, Confalonieri M et al (2000) The appropriate setting of noninvasive pressure support ventilation in stable COPD patients. Chest 118(5):1286–1293

Vitacca M, Barbano L, D'Anna S et al (2002) Comparison of five bilevel pressure ventilators in patients with chronic ventilatory failure: a physiologic study. Chest 122(6):2105–2114

Vitacca M, Bianchi L, Zanotti E et al (2004) Assessment of physiologic variables and subjective comfort under different levels of pressure support ventilation. Chest 126(3):851–859

Weaver TE, Maislin G, Dinges DF et al (2007) Relationship between hours of CPAP use and achieving normal levels of sleepiness and daily functioning. Sleep 30(6):711–719

Young T, Peppard PE, Gottlieb DJ (2002) Epidemiology of obstructive sleep apnea: a population health perspective. Am J Respir Crit Care Med 165(9):1217–1239